Quick and Easy High Protein Plant Based cookbook for everyone

Over 400 Gluten Free, Dairy Free, Low Oil and Low Salt vegetarian Recipes for Everyday Meal for Healthy Lifestyle with 30 day meal plan

Raimondi Hayden

ISBN: 9798883786227

DEDICATION
For as many who are ready to transform their diet experience without compromising on health

TABLE OF CONTENTS

INTRODUCTION

In this cookbook, you will embark on a culinary adventure that celebrates the vibrant flavors and nourishing benefits of plant-based eating. Whether you're a seasoned plant-based eater, exploring gluten-free and dairy-free options, or simply looking to incorporate more wholesome meals into your diet, this cookbook has something for everyone.

The goal is to inspire you to create delicious dishes that not only tantalize your taste buds but also support your overall health and well-being. By focusing on high-protein plant-based recipes that are free from gluten, dairy, salt, and oil, the aim is to provide you with nutritious and satisfying meals that fuel your body and nourish your soul.

Throughout this journey, this book will share essential tips and techniques for cooking without gluten, dairy, salt, and oil, empowering you to unleash your creativity in the kitchen while embracing a healthier lifestyle. From hearty breakfasts to satisfying mains, vibrant salads to decadent desserts, and everything in between, each recipe is thoughtfully crafted to showcase the incredible diversity and versatility of plant-based ingredients.

So, whether you're whipping up a quick and easy weeknight meal, hosting a gathering with friends and family, or indulging in a special treat, I hope these recipes inspire you to savor every bite and revel in the joy of nourishing your body with wholesome, plant-powered goodness.

Get ready to embark on a journey of flavor, nutrition, and culinary delight. Let's cook up something delicious together and make every meal a celebration of health and vitality!

Understanding High-Protein Plant-Based Eating

Understanding high-protein plant-based eating is essential for individuals looking to adopt a nutritious and sustainable dietary lifestyle. Below is brief overview of what high-protein plant-based eating entails:

Plant-Based Protein Sources: Contrary to common misconceptions, plant-based diets can provide ample protein through a variety of sources. These include legumes (such as beans, lentils, and chickpeas), tofu, tempeh, edamame, seitan, soy products, quinoa, nuts, seeds, and certain vegetables like spinach and broccoli. Incorporating a diverse range of these protein-rich foods into your meals ensures you meet your daily protein needs.

Complete vs. Incomplete Proteins: While animal products contain all nine essential amino acids, some plant-based protein sources lack one or more of these amino acids. However, by combining different plant-based protein sources throughout the day, such as beans and rice or hummus and whole grain bread, you can easily obtain all the essential amino acids your body needs.

Protein Requirements: The recommended dietary allowance (RDA) for protein varies depending on factors such as age, sex, weight, and activity level. Generally, adult men and women need around 0.8 grams of protein per kilogram of body weight per day. However, athletes, pregnant or breastfeeding individuals, and older adults may require higher protein intake. By choosing a variety of high-protein plant foods, you can meet your protein needs while enjoying a balanced and satisfying diet.

Benefits of Plant-Based Protein: Plant-based protein sources offer numerous health benefits, including being lower in saturated fat and cholesterol compared to animal products. Additionally, they are rich in fiber, vitamins, minerals, and phytonutrients, which contribute to overall health and well-being. Plant-based diets have been associated with lower rates of chronic diseases such as heart disease, diabetes, and certain cancers, making them a nutritious and sustainable choice for long-term health.

Balancing Macronutrients: In addition to protein, it's important to consume adequate carbohydrates and healthy fats to support overall health and energy levels. Incorporating whole grains, fruits, vegetables, nuts, seeds, and plant-based oils into your meals ensures a well-rounded and balanced diet. Experimenting with different recipes and meal combinations can help you discover delicious and satisfying ways to meet your nutritional needs while embracing plant-based eating.

Understanding the principles of high-protein plant-based eating and incorporating a variety of nutrient-dense foods into your diet, will help you to enjoy the benefits of a sustainable, flavorful, and health-promoting lifestyle. Whether you're aiming to improve your health, reduce your environmental footprint, or simply explore new culinary horizons, plant-based eating offers a world of possibilities for nourishing your body and nourishing your soul.

COOKING TIPS

Cooking without gluten, dairy, salt, and oil can seem challenging at first, but with the right tips and techniques, it can be both delicious and nutritious. Below are some tips to help you navigate gluten-free, dairy-free, salt-free, and oil-free cooking:

1. Focus on Whole Foods: Emphasize whole, unprocessed foods such as fruits, vegetables, whole grains, legumes, nuts, and seeds. These foods are naturally gluten-free, dairy-free, and low in sodium and can form the basis of many flavorful and satisfying meals.

2. Experiment with Alternative Flours: Explore gluten-free flours such as almond flour, coconut flour, rice flour, quinoa flour, and chickpea flour for baking and cooking. These flours can add texture and flavor to your dishes without gluten.

3. Use Nutritional Yeast for Flavor: Nutritional yeast is a vegan-friendly seasoning that adds a savory, cheesy flavor to dishes without the need for dairy. It's a great alternative to cheese in recipes and can be sprinkled on popcorn, salads, and pasta dishes.

4. Opt for Homemade Sauces and Dressings: Make your own sauces, dressings, and condiments using whole ingredients like fresh herbs, citrus juices, vinegar, tahini, and mustard. This allows you to control the ingredients and avoid added salt, oil, and preservatives found in store-bought versions.

5. Enhance Flavor with Herbs and Spices: Experiment with herbs, spices, and aromatic vegetables like garlic, onion, ginger, and peppers to add depth and complexity to your dishes. These natural flavor enhancers can help compensate for the absence of salt and oil.

6. **Use Citrus Juices and Vinegars:** Citrus juices (lemon, lime, orange) and vinegars (balsamic, apple cider, rice) can add brightness and acidity to dishes, enhancing flavor without the need for salt or oil. They're great for marinating proteins, dressing salads, and adding zing to sauces and soups.

7. **Explore Salt-Free Seasoning Blends:** Look for salt-free seasoning blends or make your own at home using herbs, spices, and dried aromatics. These blends can add complexity and depth of flavor to your dishes without the need for salt.

8. **Sauté with Vegetable Broth or Water:** Instead of using oil for sautéing, try using vegetable broth, water, or citrus juice to prevent sticking and add moisture to your dishes. This technique helps to reduce added fats while keeping your food flavorful and tender.

9. **Experiment with Alternative Cooking Methods:** Explore alternative cooking methods such as steaming, roasting, baking, grilling, and slow cooking to achieve delicious results without the need for oil. These methods can help retain moisture and enhance natural flavors in your food.

10. **Read Labels Carefully:** When purchasing packaged or processed foods, read labels carefully to avoid hidden sources of gluten, dairy, salt, and oil. Look for certified gluten-free, dairy-free, and low-sodium options, and choose products made with whole, natural ingredients whenever possible.

Incorporating these tips into your cooking routine, you can create flavorful, nutritious, and satisfying meals that are free from gluten, dairy, salt, and oil. With a little creativity and experimentation, you'll discover a world of delicious possibilities that support your health and well-being.

GROCERY SHOPPING TIPS AND BUDGET-FRIENDLY IDEAS

Shopping for a high-protein, gluten-free, dairy-free, oil-free, and salt-free diet can be challenging but with the right approach and some budget-friendly ideas, it's definitely manageable. Below are some tips and ideas to help you in grocery shopping:

1. Before heading to the grocery store, make a meal plan for the week. This will help you focus on what ingredients you need and prevent impulse purchases.

2. **Stick to the Perimeter:** In most grocery stores, the perimeter is where you'll find fresh produce, meats, and dairy alternatives. These whole foods will be the foundation of your diet.

3. **Read Labels:** Be diligent about reading labels to ensure products are gluten-free, dairy-free, and low in salt. Look for items specifically labeled as such or those with minimal ingredients.

4. Buy in Bulk: Purchase items like beans, lentils, quinoa, rice, nuts, and seeds in bulk. They're often cheaper this way and can be versatile sources of protein in your meals.

5 **Shop Seasonally:** Seasonal fruits and vegetables are often cheaper and fresher. Plus, they add variety to your diet.

6. **Utilize Frozen Produce:** Frozen fruits and vegetables are often just as nutritious as fresh ones and can be more budget-friendly, especially when certain items are out of season.

7. **Consider Plant-Based Proteins:** Beans, lentils, chickpeas, tofu, tempeh, and edamame are excellent sources of protein for those following a plant-based diet.

8. **Opt for Homemade:** Pre-packaged gluten-free, dairy-free, and salt-free products can be expensive. Whenever possible, make your own sauces, dressings, and snacks at home.

9. **Look for Sales and Coupons:** Keep an eye out for sales and coupons on items that fit your dietary needs. Many grocery stores offer discounts on gluten-free and dairy-free products.

10 **Stick to the Basics:** Focus on whole, unprocessed foods like fruits, vegetables, lean meats, fish, nuts, seeds, and gluten-free grains like quinoa and brown rice.

Tips for Batch cooking

Batch cooking and meal prep are excellent strategies for saving time, money, and effort in the kitchen, especially for those with dietary restrictions like a high-protein, gluten-free, dairy-free, oil-free, and salt-free diet. Below are some strategies to help you get started with Batch cooking:

1. **Plan Your Meals:** Start by planning your meals for the week. Consider your dietary restrictions and choose recipes that fit your needs.

Look for recipes that are easily adaptable to batch cooking, such as soups, stews, casseroles, and grain bowls.

2. **Make a Shopping List:** Based on your meal plan, create a detailed shopping list of all the ingredients you'll need for the week.

Try to buy ingredients in bulk when possible to save money.

3. **Prep Ingredients Ahead of Time:** Spend some time prepping ingredients in advance, such as chopping vegetables, cooking grains, and prepping proteins.

Store prepped ingredients in airtight containers or zip-top bags in the refrigerator to keep them fresh.

4. **Batch Cook Proteins:** Cook a large batch of protein sources like beans, lentils, tofu, or chicken at the beginning of the week.

Divide cooked proteins into individual portions and store them in the refrigerator or freezer for easy use in meals throughout the week.

5. **Cook Grains and Starches in Bulk:** Cook a big batch of gluten-free grains like quinoa, brown rice, or millet to use as the base for meals.

Portion out cooked grains into meal-sized containers for quick and easy meal assembly.

6. **Prepare Sauces and Dressings:** Make homemade sauces, dressings, and marinades in advance and store them in the refrigerator. Having these on hand will add flavor to your meals without relying on oil or salt.

7. **Utilize Freezer-Friendly Meals:** Prepare freezer-friendly meals like soups, stews, casseroles, and veggie burgers in large batches. Portion out these meals into individual servings and freeze them for future use.

8. **Invest in Storage Containers**: Invest in a variety of reusable storage containers in different sizes to store prepped ingredients and meals. Glass or BPA-free plastic containers are ideal for storing food safely.

9. **Label and Date Everything**: Label containers with the contents and date of preparation to help you keep track of what's in your refrigerator and freezer. Use masking tape and a permanent marker for easy labeling.

10. **Schedule Your Meal Prep Time**: Set aside dedicated time each week for meal prep. This could be a few hours on the weekend or a weekday evening. Make it a routine to ensure that you consistently have healthy meals ready to go throughout the week.

Following these batch cooking and meal prep strategies, you can streamline your cooking process, save time during busy weekdays, and ensure that you always have delicious and nutritious meals that meet your dietary needs on hand.

Tips to STAY HEALTHY AND BALANCED

Staying healthy and balanced on a plant-based diet requires careful attention to nutrient intake, variety, and portion sizes. Below are some tips to help you maintain optimal health while following a plant-based diet:

1. **Focus on Whole Foods**: Emphasize whole, minimally processed plant foods such as fruits, vegetables, whole grains, legumes, nuts, and seeds. These foods are rich in vitamins, minerals, fiber, and phytonutrients.

2. **Include a Variety of Foods**: Aim to eat a diverse range of plant foods to ensure you get a wide array of nutrients. Different plant foods offer different nutrients, so incorporating variety is key to meeting your nutritional needs.

3. **Ensure Adequate Protein Intake:** Protein is essential for overall health, and it's important to include sources of plant-based protein in your diet such as beans, lentils, tofu, tempeh, edamame, quinoa, nuts, and seeds. Combining different plant protein sources throughout the day can help ensure you get all the essential amino acids your body needs.

4. **Pay Attention to Calcium**: Calcium is important for bone health, and while dairy products are a common source, there are plenty of plant-based sources of calcium as well. Include foods like fortified plant milks, tofu, tempeh, leafy greens (such as kale and collard greens), almonds, and chia seeds in your diet.

5. **Get Enough Iron:** Iron is crucial for transporting oxygen in the blood, and plant-based sources of iron include beans, lentils, tofu, tempeh, fortified cereals, spinach, pumpkin seeds, and quinoa. Consuming vitamin C-rich foods (such as citrus fruits, bell peppers, and strawberries) alongside iron-rich foods can enhance iron absorption.

6. **Don't Forget About Omega-3 Fatty Acids**: Omega-3 fatty acids are important for heart and brain health. While fatty fish is a common source, plant-based sources include flaxseeds, chia seeds, hemp seeds, walnuts, and algae-based supplements.

7. **Be Mindful of Vitamin B12:** Vitamin B12 is primarily found in animal products, so it's important for those following a plant-based diet to supplement or consume fortified foods such as plant-based milk, nutritional yeast or breakfast cereals.

8. **Monitor Your Vitamin D Levels**: Vitamin D is important for bone health and immune function. While sunlight is a natural source, it may be challenging to get enough through sunlight alone, especially in certain climates or during winter months. Consider supplementation or consuming fortified foods like plant-based milk.

9. **Stay Hydrated**: Drink plenty of water throughout the day to stay hydrated, as water is essential for digestion, nutrient absorption, and overall health.

10. **Practice Portion Control**: While plant-based foods are generally lower in calories compared to animal products, portion control is still important to maintain a healthy weight and balance nutrient intake.

11. **Consider Consulting a Registered Dietitian:** If you're new to a plant-based diet or have specific health concerns, consider consulting a registered dietitian who specializes in plant-based nutrition. They can help you create a balanced meal plan tailored to your individual needs and provide guidance on meeting your nutritional requirements.

Following these tips and ensuring a well-rounded, plant-based diet, you can maintain optimal health and wellness while enjoying the benefits of plant-based eating.

30 DAYS MEAL PLAN

Day 1:

Breakfast: Quinoa Breakfast Bowl topped with sliced bananas, chopped nuts (such as almonds or walnuts), and a drizzle of almond milk.

Lunch: Chickpea Salad with mixed greens, cherry tomatoes, cucumber slices, bell pepper strips, and a lemon-tahini dressing.

Dinner: Lentil Soup with diced vegetables (carrots, celery, onions), garlic, vegetable broth, and herbs (thyme, rosemary, parsley).

Snack: Sliced apples with almond butter.

Day 2:

Breakfast: Protein Smoothie made with mixed berries, spinach, plant-based protein powder, almond milk, and chia seeds.

Lunch: Stuffed Bell Peppers filled with a mixture of cooked quinoa, black beans, corn, diced tomatoes, and spices.

Dinner: Grilled Tofu with Roasted Vegetables (broccoli, cauliflower, carrots) seasoned with lemon juice, garlic, and herbs.

Snack: Raw Veggie Sticks (carrots, cucumber, bell pepper) with homemade hummus.

Day 3:

Breakfast: Chia Seed Pudding made with coconut milk, vanilla extract, and topped with fresh berries.

Lunch: Quinoa Salad with mixed greens, cherry tomatoes, diced cucumber, avocado slices, and a lemon-tahini dressing.

Dinner: Baked Portobello Mushrooms stuffed with a mixture of quinoa, spinach, onions, and garlic.

Snack: Rice cakes with mashed avocado and cherry tomatoes.

Day 4:
Breakfast: Smoothie Bowl topped with sliced banana, shredded coconut, and a sprinkle of hemp seeds.
Lunch: Lentil and Vegetable Stir-Fry with broccoli, bell peppers, snap peas, and a gluten-free tamari sauce.
Dinner: Chickpea and Vegetable Curry served over brown rice, flavored with coconut milk, curry powder, and turmeric.
Snack: Trail mix made with almonds, pumpkin seeds, and dried fruit.

Day 5:
Breakfast: Overnight Oats made with gluten-free oats, almond milk, chia seeds, and topped with sliced strawberries and a drizzle of maple syrup.
Lunch: Spinach and Strawberry Salad with sliced almonds, avocado, and a balsamic vinaigrette.
Dinner: Quinoa and Black Bean Enchiladas made with corn tortillas, homemade enchilada sauce, and topped with avocado slices.
Snack: Apple slices with almond butter.

Day 6:
Breakfast: Banana Walnut Pancakes made with mashed banana, almond flour, flaxseed meal, and topped with chopped walnuts.
Lunch: Mediterranean Chickpea Salad with diced cucumbers, cherry tomatoes, red onion, kalamata olives, and a lemon-tahini dressing.
Dinner: Baked Sweet Potato topped with black beans, salsa, avocado, and chopped cilantro.
Snack: Veggie sticks with salt-free guacamole.

Day 7:
Breakfast: Tofu Scramble with sautéed vegetables (bell peppers, onions, spinach) and served with gluten-free toast.
Lunch: Quinoa and Vegetable Soup with diced carrots, celery, zucchini, and vegetable broth.
Dinner: Stir-Fried Tofu and Mixed Vegetables with brown rice, flavored with garlic, ginger, and gluten-free tamari sauce.
Snack: Rice cakes with mashed avocado and sliced cucumber.

Day 8:
Breakfast: Quinoa Porridge made with cooked quinoa, almond milk, sliced bananas, and chopped nuts.
Lunch: Lentil Salad with mixed greens, cooked lentils, cherry tomatoes, cucumber slices, and a lemon-tahini dressing.
Dinner: Baked Tofu with Roasted Vegetables (such as broccoli, cauliflower, and carrots) seasoned with herbs and lemon juice.
Snack: Sliced apples with almond butter.

Day 9:
Breakfast: Protein Smoothie made with mixed berries, spinach, plant-based protein powder, and almond milk.
Lunch: Chickpea and Vegetable Stir-Fry with bell peppers, snap peas, carrots, and gluten-free tamari sauce.
Dinner: Stuffed Bell Peppers filled with quinoa, black beans, corn, diced tomatoes, and spices.

Snack: Raw Veggie Sticks (carrots, cucumber, bell pepper) with homemade hummus.
Day 10:
Breakfast: Chia Seed Pudding made with coconut milk, chia seeds, and topped with sliced strawberries.
Lunch: Quinoa and Black Bean Salad with diced avocado, cherry tomatoes, red onion, and a lime-cilantro dressing.
Dinner: Lentil and Vegetable Curry served over brown rice, flavored with coconut milk, curry powder, and turmeric.
Snack: Rice cakes with mashed avocado and cherry tomatoes.
Day 11:
Breakfast: Smoothie Bowl topped with sliced banana, shredded coconut, and a sprinkle of hemp seeds.
Lunch: Spinach and Strawberry Salad with sliced almonds, avocado, and a balsamic vinaigrette.
Dinner: Portobello Mushroom Burgers served on lettuce wraps with tomato slices, avocado, and mustard.
Snack: Trail mix made with almonds, pumpkin seeds, and dried fruit.
Day 12:
Breakfast: Buckwheat Pancakes made with buckwheat flour, flaxseed meal, almond milk, and topped with fresh berries.
Lunch: Mediterranean Chickpea Salad with diced cucumbers, kalamata olives, red onion, and a lemon-tahini dressing.
Dinner: Quinoa and Vegetable Soup with carrots, celery, zucchini, and vegetable broth.
Snack: Apple slices with almond butter.
Day 13:
Breakfast: Tofu Scramble with sautéed vegetables (bell peppers, onions, spinach) and gluten-free toast.
Lunch: Mixed Bean Salad with kidney beans, black beans, chickpeas, diced bell peppers, and a lemon-tahini dressing.
Dinner: Baked Sweet Potato topped with black beans, salsa, avocado, and chopped cilantro.
Snack: Veggie sticks with salt-free guacamole.
Day 14:
Breakfast: Overnight Oats made with gluten-free oats, almond milk, chia seeds, and topped with sliced bananas and a drizzle of maple syrup.
Lunch: Quinoa and Kale Salad with diced tomatoes, cucumber slices, avocado, and a lemon-tahini dressing.
Dinner: Stir-Fried Tempeh and Mixed Vegetables with brown rice, flavored with garlic, ginger, and gluten-free tamari sauce.
Snack: Rice cakes with mashed avocado and sliced cucumber.
Day 15:
Breakfast: Quinoa Porridge topped with mixed berries, sliced almonds, and a drizzle of maple syrup.
Lunch: Lentil and Vegetable Soup with a side of gluten-free crackers or bread.
Dinner: Baked Tofu with Steamed Broccoli and a side of quinoa.

Snack: Sliced apples with almond butter.

Day 16:
Breakfast: Chia Seed Pudding made with coconut milk, topped with sliced bananas and chopped walnuts.
Lunch: Chickpea Salad with mixed greens, cherry tomatoes, cucumber slices, and a lemon-tahini dressing.
Dinner: Stuffed Bell Peppers filled with quinoa, black beans, corn, and diced tomatoes.
Snack: Carrot sticks with hummus.

Day 17:
Breakfast: Protein Smoothie made with mixed berries, spinach, hemp seeds, and almond milk.
Lunch: Quinoa and Black Bean Salad with diced avocado, red onion, cilantro, and a lime-cumin dressing.
Dinner: Lentil Bolognese served over gluten-free pasta or spiralized zucchini noodles.
Snack: Rice cakes with mashed avocado and cherry tomatoes.

Day 18:
Breakfast: Buckwheat Pancakes topped with sliced strawberries and a drizzle of agave syrup.
Lunch: Spinach and Strawberry Salad with sliced almonds, avocado, and a balsamic vinaigrette.
Dinner: Portobello Mushroom Burgers served on lettuce wraps with tomato slices and mashed avocado.
Snack: Trail mix made with almonds, pumpkin seeds, and dried fruit.

Day 19:
Breakfast: Smoothie Bowl topped with sliced banana, shredded coconut, and granola.
Lunch: Mediterranean Chickpea Salad with diced cucumber, kalamata olives, red onion, and a lemon-tahini dressing.
Dinner: Quinoa Stir-Fry with mixed vegetables (bell peppers, snap peas, carrots) and tofu, seasoned with gluten-free tamari sauce.
Snack: Apple slices with almond butter.

Day 20:
Breakfast: Tofu Scramble with sautéed vegetables (bell peppers, onions, spinach) and gluten-free toast.
Lunch: Mixed Bean Salad with kidney beans, black beans, chickpeas, diced bell peppers, and a lemon-tahini dressing.
Dinner: Baked Sweet Potato topped with black beans, salsa, avocado, and chopped cilantro.
Snack: Veggie sticks with salt-free guacamole.

Day 21:
Breakfast: Overnight Oats made with gluten-free oats, almond milk, chia seeds, and topped with sliced peaches and a sprinkle of cinnamon.
Lunch: Quinoa and Kale Salad with diced tomatoes, cucumber slices, avocado, and a lemon-tahini dressing.

Dinner: Stir-Fried Tempeh and Mixed Vegetables with brown rice, flavored with garlic, ginger, and gluten-free tamari sauce.

Snack: Rice cakes with mashed avocado and sliced cucumber.

Day 22:

Breakfast: Tofu Scramble with sautéed spinach, mushrooms, and onions, seasoned with turmeric, garlic powder, and nutritional yeast.

Lunch: Quinoa and Black Bean Salad with diced bell peppers, cherry tomatoes, avocado, and a lime-cilantro dressing.

Dinner: Lentil Soup with mixed vegetables (carrots, celery, kale) and herbs (thyme, rosemary, bay leaves).

Snack: Sliced apple with almond butter.

Day 23:

Breakfast: Protein Smoothie made with banana, frozen berries, spinach, hemp seeds, and unsweetened almond milk.

Lunch: Chickpea and Vegetable Stir-Fry with broccoli, bell peppers, snap peas, and gluten-free tamari sauce.

Dinner: Baked Portobello Mushrooms stuffed with quinoa, diced tomatoes, garlic, and herbs.

Snack: Carrot sticks with hummus.

Day 24:

Breakfast: Overnight Chia Seed Pudding made with chia seeds, almond milk, vanilla extract, and topped with sliced strawberries.

Lunch: Spinach Salad with sliced almonds, dried cranberries, avocado, and a lemon-tahini dressing.

Dinner: Lentil and Vegetable Curry served over brown rice, flavored with coconut milk, curry powder, and turmeric.

Snack: Rice cakes with mashed avocado and cherry tomatoes.

Day 25:

Breakfast: Buckwheat Pancakes topped with mixed berries and a drizzle of pure maple syrup.

Lunch: Quinoa Salad with diced cucumber, cherry tomatoes, red onion, olives, and a balsamic vinaigrette.

Dinner: Stuffed Bell Peppers filled with black beans, corn, diced tomatoes, and cilantro.

Snack: Trail mix made with almonds, pumpkin seeds, and dried fruit.

Day 26:

Breakfast: Smoothie Bowl topped with sliced banana, shredded coconut, and gluten-free granola.

Lunch: Mediterranean Chickpea Salad with diced cucumber, cherry tomatoes, red onion, kalamata olives, and a lemon-tahini dressing.

Dinner: Tofu and Vegetable Stir-Fry with snow peas, carrots, bell peppers, and a homemade teriyaki sauce.

Snack: Apple slices with almond butter.

Day 27:

Breakfast: Quinoa Breakfast Bowl with cooked quinoa, almond milk, chopped nuts, and diced apples.

Lunch: Lentil and Vegetable Soup with gluten-free crackers or bread.

Dinner: Baked Sweet Potato topped with black beans, salsa, avocado, and cilantro.
Snack: Veggie sticks with salt-free guacamole.
Day 28:
Breakfast: Chia Seed Pudding made with coconut milk, topped with sliced bananas and a sprinkle of cinnamon.
Lunch: Mixed Bean Salad with kidney beans, black beans, chickpeas, diced bell peppers, and a lemon-tahini dressing.
Dinner: Quinoa Stir-Fry with mixed vegetables (broccoli, cauliflower, carrots) and tofu, seasoned with gluten-free tamari sauce.
Snack: Rice cakes with mashed avocado and sliced cucumber.
Day 29:
Breakfast: Protein Smoothie made with mixed berries, spinach, plant-based protein powder, almond milk, and chia seeds.
Lunch: Quinoa and Kale Salad with diced tomatoes, cucumber slices, avocado, and a lemon-tahini dressing.
Dinner: Grilled Tofu with Roasted Vegetables (broccoli, cauliflower, carrots) seasoned with lemon juice, garlic, and herbs.
Snack: Raw Veggie Sticks (carrots, cucumber, bell pepper) with homemade hummus.
Day 30:
Breakfast: Chia Seed Pudding made with coconut milk, topped with sliced bananas and chopped walnuts.
Lunch: Quinoa Salad with mixed greens, cherry tomatoes, diced cucumber, avocado slices, and a lemon-tahini dressing.
Dinner: Baked Sweet Potato topped with black beans, salsa, avocado, and chopped cilantro.
Snack: Rice cakes with mashed avocado and cherry tomatoes.
Feel free to adjust the portion sizes and ingredients to fit your preferences and dietary needs. This meal plan provides a variety of nutritious and satisfying meals while adhering to a high-protein, plant-based, gluten-free, dairy-free, oil-free, and salt-free diet.

BREAKFAST RECIPES

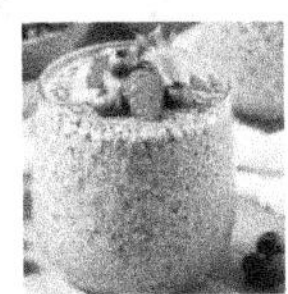

Protein-Packed Chia Pudding

Creamy and satisfying chia seed pudding infused with plant-based protein.
Preparation Time: 5 minutes, Total Time: 4 hours (for chilling), serving: 2
Ingredients: 1/4 cup chia seeds, 1 cup unsweetened almond milk, 2 tablespoons maple syrup, 1 scoop plant-based protein powder, fresh berries for topping
Directions:

1. In a bowl, whisk together chia seeds, almond milk, maple syrup, and plant-based protein powder.
2. Let it sit for 5 minutes, then whisk again to prevent clumping.
3. Cover the bowl and refrigerate for at least 4 hours or overnight, until the pudding thickens.
4. Serve chilled, topped with fresh berries.
Nutritional Info: Calories: 220, Protein: 15g, Fat: 8g, Carbohydrates: 20g

Breakfast Tacos

These tacos are perfect for a hearty breakfast, filled with tofu scramble and black beans.
Preparation Time: 15 minutes, Cooking Time: 15 minutes, Total Time: 30 minutes, serving: 4
Ingredients: 8 corn tortillas, 1 block tofu (pressed and crumbled), 1 cup cooked black beans, 1 cup diced bell peppers, 1 cup diced tomatoes, 1/2 cup diced onions, 1 teaspoon garlic powder, 1/2 teaspoon paprika, 1 teaspoon turmeric, 1/4 teaspoon black pepper.
Direction:
1. In a skillet, sauté onions, bell peppers, and tomatoes until softened.
2. Add crumbled tofu and spices and cook until heated through.
3. Warm tortillas and fill with tofu scramble and black beans and Serve immediately.
Nutritional Info: Calories: 180, Protein: 10g, Fat: 5g, Carbohydrates: 25g

Tofu Breakfast Burritos

Flavorful breakfast burritos filled with seasoned tofu scramble and fresh vegetables.
Preparation Time: 10 minutes, Cooking Time: 10 minutes, Total Time: 20 minutes, serving: 2
Ingredients: 1/2 block (7 oz) firm tofu, crumbled, 1/2 cup diced bell peppers, 1/2 cup chopped spinach, 2 whole grain gluten-free tortillas, 1/4 cup salsa, 1/2 avocado, sliced,Fresh cilantro for garnish
Directions:
1. In a skillet over medium heat, sauté crumbled tofu, bell peppers, and spinach until tofu is lightly browned and vegetables are tender.
2. Warm tortillas in the skillet or microwave.
3. Divide tofu scramble evenly between the tortillas.
4. Top with salsa, sliced avocado, and fresh cilantro.
5. Roll up the tortillas into burritos and serve warm.
Nutritional Info: Calories: 290, Protein: 15g, Fat: 12g, Carbohydrates: 30g

Vegan Protein Pancakes

Fluffy pancakes made with chickpea flour and plant-based protein powder.
Preparation Time: 10 minutes, Cooking Time: 10 minutes, Total Time: 20 minutes, Serving: 2

Ingredients: 1 cup chickpea flour, 1 scoop plant-based protein powder, 1 tsp baking powder, 1/2 cup unsweetened almond milk, 1 ripe banana, mashed, Fresh berries for topping

Directions:

1. In a bowl, whisk together chickpea flour, plant-based protein powder, and baking powder.
2. Stir in almond milk and mashed banana until smooth.
3. Heat a non-stick skillet over medium heat and lightly grease with cooking spray.
4. Pour 1/4 cup of batter onto the skillet for each pancake.
5. Cook for 2-3 minutes until bubbles form on the surface, then flip and cook for another 2-3 minutes until golden brown.
6. Serve warm, topped with fresh berries.

Nutritional Info: Calories: 280, Protein: 20g, Fat: 8g, Carbohydrates: 35g

Vegan Breakfast Bowl

Wholesome breakfast bowl featuring quinoa, mixed vegetables, and tofu scramble.

Preparation Time: 10 minutes, Cooking Time: 15 minutes, Total Time: 25 minutes, Serving: 2

Ingredients: 1/2 cup uncooked quinoa, 1 cup water or vegetable broth, 1/2 block (7 oz) firm tofu, crumbled, 1/2 cup diced bell peppers, 1/2 cup cherry tomatoes, halved, 2 cups baby spinach, 1/2 avocado, sliced, Fresh parsley for garnish

Directions:

1. Rinse quinoa under cold water, then combine with water or vegetable broth in a saucepan.
2. Bring to a boil, then reduce heat, cover, and simmer for 15 minutes until quinoa is cooked and liquid is absorbed.
3. In a skillet over medium heat, sauté crumbled tofu, bell peppers, cherry tomatoes, and baby spinach until vegetables are tender.
4. Divide cooked quinoa and tofu scramble between bowls.
5. Top with sliced avocado and fresh parsley.
6. Serve warm and enjoy!

Nutritional Info: Calories: 320, Protein: 18g, Fat: 14g, Carbohydrates: 35g

Vegan Breakfast Smoothie

Energizing smoothie blended with banana, spinach, almond butter, and plant-based protein powder.

Preparation Time: 5 minutes, Total Time: 5 minutes, Serving: 1

Ingredients: 1 ripe banana, 1 cup fresh spinach, 1 tbsp almond butter, 1 scoop plant-based protein powder, 1 cup unsweetened almond milk, Ice cubes (optional)

Directions:

1. In a blender, combine banana, spinach, almond butter, plant-based protein powder, and almond milk.
2. Blend until smooth and creamy.
3. Add ice cubes if desired and blend again until smooth.
4. Pour into a glass and enjoy immediately.

Nutritional Info: Calories: 290, Protein: 20g, Fat: 10g, Carbohydrates: 30g

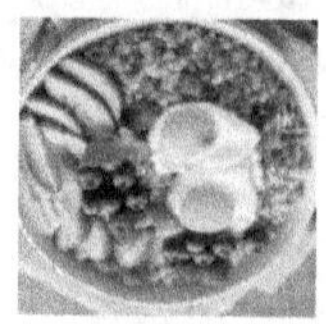

Quinoa and berries Breakfast Bowl

A hearty and nutritious breakfast bowl featuring protein-rich quinoa, fresh fruits, nuts, and seeds.
Preparation Time: 10 minutes Cooking Time: 15 minutes Total Time: 25 minutes Serving Size: 2
Ingredients: 1 cup cooked quinoa 1 ripe banana, sliced, 1/2 cup fresh berries (such as strawberries, blueberries, or raspberries), 2 tablespoons chopped nuts (such as almonds or walnuts), 1 tablespoon chia seeds, 1 tablespoon hemp seeds, 1 tablespoon agave nectar or maple syrup (optional)
Directions:
1. In a bowl, divide cooked quinoa evenly.
2. Top with sliced banana, fresh berries, chopped nuts, chia seeds, and hemp seeds.
3. Drizzle with maple syrup or agave nectar if desired.
4. Serve immediately and enjoy!
Nutritional Info (per serving): Calories: 300 Protein: 10g Carbohydrates: 50g Fat: 8g Fiber: 8g

Vegan Chickpea Flour Pancakes

Fluffy and protein-packed pancakes made with chickpea flour, perfect for a satisfying breakfast.
Preparation Time: 10 minutes Cooking Time: 10 minutes Total Time: 20 minutes, Serving Size: 4 pancakes
Ingredients: 1 cup chickpea flour, 1 teaspoon baking powder, 1 tablespoon ground flaxseed mixed with 3 tablespoons water (as an egg substitute), 1/2 cup almond milk, 1 tablespoon maple syrup, 1/2 teaspoon vanilla extract
Directions:
1. In a bowl, whisk together chickpea flour and baking powder.
2. In a separate bowl, mix together flaxseed mixture, almond milk, maple syrup, and vanilla extract.
3. Pour wet ingredients into dry ingredients and stir until well combined.
4. Heat a non-stick skillet over medium heat and pour 1/4 cup of batter for each pancake.
5. Cook for 2-3 minutes on each side until golden brown.
6. Serve warm with your favorite toppings and enjoy!
Nutritional Info (per serving): Calories: 200 Protein: 12g Carbohydrates: 25g Fat: 7g Fiber: 5g

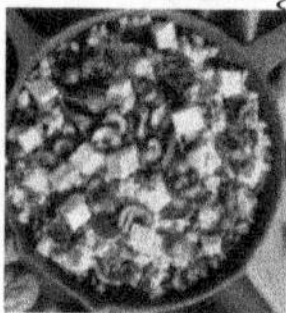

Tofu Scramble with Spinach and Mushrooms

A savory and protein-rich scramble made with tofu, spinach, and mushrooms, seasoned with herbs and spices.

Preparation Time: 10 minutes, Cooking Time: 15 minutes Total Time: 25 minutes
Serving Size: 2

Ingredients:

1 block firm tofu, drained and crumbled
1 cup chopped spinach
1 cup sliced mushrooms
1/2 onion, diced
2 cloves garlic, minced
1/2 teaspoon turmeric powder
1/2 teaspoon cumin powder
Salt and pepper to taste
Fresh parsley or cilantro for garnish

Directions:

1. In a skillet, sauté onion and garlic until translucent.
2. Add sliced mushrooms and cook until softened.
3. Stir in crumbled tofu, turmeric, cumin, salt, and pepper.
4. Cook for 5-7 minutes, stirring occasionally.
5. Add the chopped spinach to the skillet and cook until wilted.
6. Serve hot, garnished with fresh parsley or cilantro.

Nutritional Info (per serving): Calories: 180 Protein: 15g Carbohydrates: 10g Fat: 9g Fiber: 3g

Chia Seed Pudding with Mixed Berries

A creamy and nutritious pudding made with chia seeds and almond milk, topped with fresh mixed berries.

Preparation Time: 5 minutes (plus chilling time), Cooking Time: 0 minutes, Total Time: 4 hours 5 minutes, Serving Size: 2

Ingredients: 1/4 cup chia seeds,1 cup unsweetened almond milk, 1 tablespoon maple syrup or agave nectar, 1/2 teaspoon vanilla extract, 1/2 cup mixed berries (such as strawberries, blueberries, and raspberries)

Directions:

1. In a bowl, whisk together chia seeds, almond milk, maple syrup, and vanilla extract. Let it sit for about 5 minutes,
2. Whisk the mixture again to prevent clumping.
3. Cover and refrigerate for at least 4 hours or overnight, until thickened.
4. Serve chilled, topped with mixed berries.

Nutritional Info (per serving): Calories: 150 Protein: 5g Carbohydrates: 20g Fat: 7g Fiber: 8g

Tofu Berry Smoothie Bowl

A refreshing and protein-packed smoothie bowl made with silken tofu and mixed berries, topped with crunchy granola and coconut flakes.

Preparation Time: 5 minutes Cooking Time: 0 minutes Total Time: 5 minutes
Serving Size: 1

Ingredients: 1/2 cup silken tofu, 1/2 cup mixed berries (fresh or frozen), 1 ripe banana, frozen, 1/4 cup unsweetened almond milk, 1 tablespoon chia seeds, Toppings: Granola, coconut flakes, sliced fruit
Directions:
1. In a blender, combine silken tofu, mixed berries, frozen banana, almond milk, and chia seeds.
2. Blend mixture until smooth and creamy, add more almond milk if needed to get the desired consistency.
3. Pour the smoothie into a bowl and top with granola, coconut flakes, and sliced fruit.
4. Serve immediately and enjoy!
Nutritional Info (per serving): Calories: 250 Protein: 12g Carbohydrates: 35g Fat: 8g Fiber: 8g

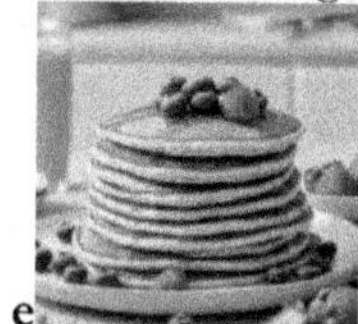

Vegan Protein Pancake Stack

A stack of fluffy protein pancakes made with oats, banana, and plant-based protein powder, perfect for a hearty breakfast.
Preparation Time: 10 minutes Cooking Time: 10 minutes Total Time: 20 minutes
Serving Size: 2
Ingredients: 1 cup rolled oats (gluten-free if necessary), 1 ripe banana, 1 scoop plant-based protein powder, 1/2 cup unsweetened almond milk, 1 teaspoon baking powder, 1/2 teaspoon vanilla extract, Toppings: Fresh fruit, nut butter, maple syrup
Directions:

1. In a blender, combine rolled oats, banana, plant-based protein powder, almond milk, baking powder, and vanilla extract.
2. Blend until smooth and creamy, adding more almond milk if needed to achieve a pourable batter consistency.
3. Heat a non-stick skillet over medium heat and pour 1/4 cup of batter for each pancake.
4. Cook for 2-3 minutes on each side until golden brown.
5. Stack the pancakes on a plate and top with your favorite toppings.
6. Serve warm and enjoy!
Nutritional Info (per serving): Calories: 300 Protein: 15g Carbohydrates: 45g Fat: 7g Fiber: 6g

Almond Butter Banana Breakfast Cookies

These chewy and satisfying breakfast cookies are made with almond butter, bananas, and oats, making them a perfect on-the-go option.
Preparation Time: 10 minutes, Cooking Time: 15 minutes, Total Time: 25 minutes, Serving Size: 8 cookies

Ingredients: 1 ripe banana, mashed, 1/2 cup almond butter, 1 tablespoon maple syrup or agave nectar, 1 teaspoon vanilla extract, 1 cup rolled oats (gluten-free if necessary), 1/4 cup almond flour, 1/2 teaspoon baking powder, 1/4 cup chopped nuts or seeds (optional)

Directions:

1. Preheat the oven to 350°F (175°C) and properly line a baking sheet with parchment paper.
2. In a bowl, mix together mashed banana, almond butter, maple syrup, and vanilla extract until smooth.
3. Add rolled oats, almond flour, baking powder, and chopped nuts or seeds (if using) to the wet ingredients and mix until well combined.
4. Scoop spoonful of the dough onto the prepared baking sheet and flatten slightly with the back of a spoon.
5. Bake until cookies is golden brown around the edges, for about 12-15 minutes.
6. Allow the cookies to cool on the baking sheet for 5 minutes before transferring to a wire rack to cool completely.
7. Serve and enjoy as a delicious breakfast or snack!

Nutritional Info (per serving - 1 cookie): Calories: 150 Protein: 5g Carbohydrates: 15g Fat: 8g Fiber: 3g

Protein-Packed Green Smoothie

A refreshing and nutrient-rich green smoothie made with leafy greens, fruit, plant-based protein powder, and creamy almond milk.

Preparation Time: 5 minutes, Cooking Time: 0 minutes, Total Time: 5 minutes, Serving Size: 1

Ingredients: 1 cup unsweetened almond milk, 1 scoop plant-based protein powder (vanilla or unflavored), 1 cup fresh spinach or kale, 1/2 frozen banana, 1/2 cup frozen mixed berries, 1 tablespoon chia seeds or flaxseeds

Directions:

1. In a blender, combine almond milk, plant-based protein powder, fresh spinach or kale, frozen banana, frozen mixed berries, and chia seeds or flaxseeds.
2. Blend the mixture until smooth and creamy, add more almond milk if needed to reach desired consistency.
3. Pour into a glass and serve immediately as a nutritious breakfast or snack.

Nutritional Info (per serving): Calories: 250, Protein: 20g, Carbohydrates: 30g, Fat: 7g, Fiber: 8g

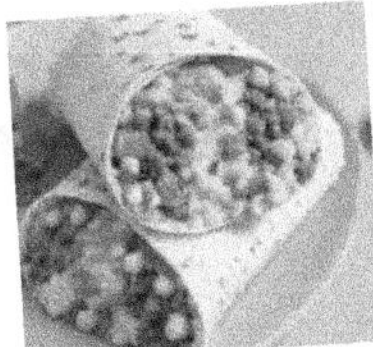

Chickpea Flour Breakfast Burrito

A protein-packed breakfast burrito filled with savory chickpea flour omelet, fresh vegetables, and creamy avocado.

Preparation Time: 10 minutes, Cooking Time: 15 minutes, Total Time: 25 minutes, Serving Size: 2
Ingredients: 1 cup chickpea flour, 1 cup water, 1/2 teaspoon baking powder, 1/2 teaspoon turmeric powder, 1/2 teaspoon garlic powder, Salt and pepper to taste, 1/2 cup diced bell peppers, 1/4 cup diced onion, 1/4 cup diced tomatoes, 1/4 cup chopped fresh cilantro, 1 ripe avocado, sliced, 2 gluten-free tortillas
Directions:
1. In a bowl, whisk together chickpea flour, water, baking powder, turmeric powder, garlic powder, salt, and pepper until smooth.
2. Heat a non-stick skillet over medium heat and pour half of the chickpea flour batter to make a thin omelet.
3. Cook for 2-3 minutes on each side until golden brown and cooked through. Repeat with the remaining batter.
4. Place the cooked chickpea flour omelets on gluten-free tortillas.
5. Top with diced bell peppers, onion, tomatoes, fresh cilantro, and sliced avocado.
6. Roll up the tortillas into burritos, slice in half if desired, and serve.
Nutritional Info (per serving): Calories: 350 Protein: 15g Carbohydrates: 40g Fat: 15g Fiber: 10g

Sweet Potato Breakfast Hash

A hearty and flavorful breakfast hash made with roasted sweet potatoes, black beans, and colorful vegetables, topped with avocado and salsa.
Preparation Time: 15 minutes, Cooking Time: 30 minutes, Total Time: 45 minutes, Serving Size: 4
Ingredients: 2 large sweet potatoes, peeled and diced, 1 tablespoon chili powder, 1 teaspoon cumin, 1/2 teaspoon paprika, Salt and pepper to taste, 1 tablespoon olive oil (optional, can omit for oil-free), 1 can black beans, drained and rinsed, 1 bell pepper, diced, 1/2 onion, diced, 2 cloves garlic, minced, 1 avocado, diced, Salsa for serving
Directions:
1. Preheat the oven to 400°F (200°C) and line a baking sheet with parchment paper.
2. In a bowl, toss diced sweet potatoes with chili powder, cumin, paprika, salt, pepper, and olive oil (if using) until evenly coated.
3. Spread the seasoned sweet potatoes in a single layer on the prepared baking sheet and roast for 25-30 minutes until tender and caramelized.
4. In a skillet, sauté bell pepper, onion, and garlic until softened.
5. Add black beans to the skillet and cook until heated through.
6. Add roasted sweet potatoes to the skillet and stir to combine.
7. Serve the breakfast hash topped with salsa and diced avocado.

Nutritional Info (per serving): Calories: 300 Protein: 10g Carbohydrates: 45g Fat: 10g Fiber: 10g

LUNCH RECIPES

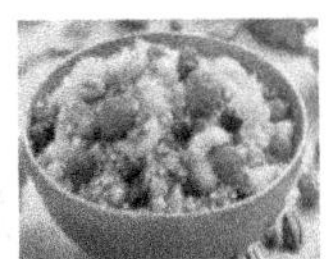

Quinoa Fruit Salad with Nuts

This refreshing salad combines protein-rich quinoa with a variety of fresh fruits and nuts for a satisfying and nutritious lunch.

Preparation Time: 10 minutes, Cooking Time: 15 minutes, Total Time: 25 minutes, Serving Size: 2

Ingredients: 1 cup cooked quinoa, 1 ripe banana, sliced, 1/2 cup fresh berries (such as strawberries, blueberries, or raspberries), 2, tablespoons chopped nuts (such as almonds or walnuts), 1 tablespoon chia seeds, 1 tablespoon hemp seeds, 1 tablespoon maple syrup or agave nectar (optional)

Directions:

1. In a large bowl, combine cooked quinoa, sliced banana, fresh berries, chopped nuts, chia seeds, and hemp seeds.
2. Drizzle with maple syrup or agave nectar if desired.
3. Toss gently until all ingredients are well combined.
4. Divide into serving bowls and enjoy this nutritious and flavorful salad!

Nutritional Info (per serving): Calories: 300 Protein: 8g Carbohydrates: 45g Fat: 10g Fiber: 7g

Chickpea and Vegetable Stir-Fry

This savory stir-fry features protein-packed chickpeas and a colorful array of vegetables, all tossed in a flavorful sauce for a quick and satisfying lunch.

Preparation Time: 10 minutes, Cooking Time: 15 minutes, Total Time: 25 minutes, Serving Size: 2

Ingredients: 1 can chickpeas, drained and rinsed, 2 cups mixed vegetables (such as bell peppers, broccoli, carrots, and snap peas), 2 cloves garlic, minced, 2 tablespoons low-sodium soy sauce (or tamari for gluten-free), 1 tablespoon rice vinegar, 1 tablespoon maple syrup, 1 teaspoon cornstarch, 2 tablespoons water

Directions:

1. In a small bowl, whisk together soy sauce, rice vinegar, maple syrup, cornstarch, and water to make the sauce. Set aside.
2. Heat a non-stick skillet over medium heat and add chickpeas. Cook for about 6 minutes or until lightly golden brown,
3. Add minced garlic and mixed vegetables to the skillet. Cook for about 5 minutes, until vegetables are tender-crisp
4. Pour the sauce over the chickpeas and vegetables. Stir well to coat everything evenly.

5. Cook until the sauce is thickens for another 3 minutes.

6. Serve hot over cooked quinoa or brown rice, if desired.

Nutritional Info (per serving without rice/quinoa): Calories: 250 Protein: 12g Carbohydrates: 35g Fat: 6g Fiber: 8g

Spinach and Lentil Salad

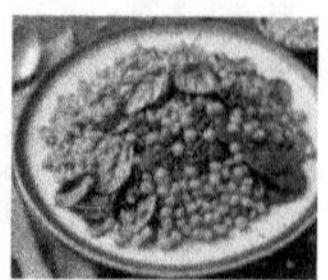

This hearty salad features protein-rich lentils, fresh spinach, and colorful vegetables, all tossed in a zesty lemon vinaigrette for a light and satisfying lunch.

Preparation Time: 10 minutes, Cooking Time: 15 minutes, Total Time: 25 minutes, Serving Size: 2

Ingredients: 1 cup cooked lentils,2 cups fresh spinach leaves, 1/2 cup cherry tomatoes, halved, 1/4 cup sliced cucumber, 1/4 cup diced red onion,2 tablespoons chopped fresh parsley, 2 tablespoons lemon juice, 1 tablespoon olive oil (optional, omit for oil-free), Salt and pepper to taste

Directions:

1. In a large bowl, combine cooked lentils, fresh spinach leaves, cherry tomatoes, cucumber, red onion, and fresh parsley.

2. In a small bowl, whisk together lemon juice, olive oil (if using), salt, and pepper to make the dressing.

3. Pour the dressing over the salad and toss gently until everything is well coated.

4. Divide into serving bowls and enjoy this nutritious and flavorful salad!

Nutritional Info (per serving): Calories: 280 Protein: 15g Carbohydrates: 35g Fat: 6g Fiber: 12g

Chickpea Buddha Bowl

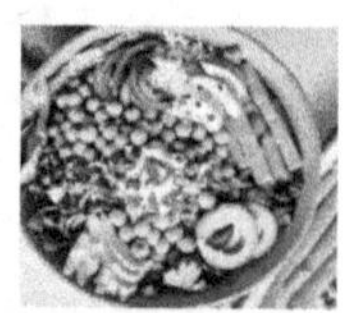

A nourishing Buddha bowl filled with protein-rich chickpeas, quinoa, roasted vegetables, and creamy avocado.

Preparation Time: 15 minutes, Cooking Time: 25 minutes, Total Time: 40 minutes, serving: 2

Ingredients: 1 can (15 oz) chickpeas, drained and rinsed, 1 cup cooked quinoa, 2 cups mixed vegetables (such as broccoli, carrots, and cauliflower), chopped, 1/2 avocado, sliced, 2 tablespoons lemon juice ,2 tablespoons tahini, 1 clove garlic, minced, Black pepper, to taste

Directions:

1. Preheat oven to 400°F (200°C). Place mixed vegetables on a baking sheet and roast for 20-25 minutes until tender.

2. In a skillet, sauté chickpeas over medium heat until lightly browned.

3. In a small bowl, whisk together lemon juice, tahini, minced garlic, and black pepper to make the dressing.
4. Divide cooked quinoa, roasted vegetables, and sautéed chickpeas into bowls.
5. Top with sliced avocado and drizzle with the tahini dressing.
6. Serve warm and enjoy!
Nutritional Info: Calories: 320, Protein: 18g, Fat: 12g, Carbohydrates: 40g

Chickpea Avocado Tacos

These tacos are a nutritious and satisfying lunch option, featuring a creamy avocado and chickpea filling.

Preparation Time: 20 minutes, Cooking Time: 10 minutes, Total Time: 30 minutes, serving: 4

Ingredients: 8 corn tortillas, 1 can chickpeas (drained and rinsed), 1 avocado (mashed), 1/4 cup diced red onion, 1/4 cup chopped cilantro, 2 tablespoons lime juice, 1/2 teaspoon cumin, 1/2 teaspoon chili powder, 1/4 teaspoon garlic powder.

Direction:

1. In a bowl, mix mashed avocado, lime juice, cumin, chili powder, and garlic powder.
2. Heat chickpeas in a skillet until warm.
3. Warm tortillas and fill with mashed avocado mixture and chickpeas.
4. Top with diced onions and cilantro.
5. Serve chickpea avocado tacos immediately and enjoy
Nutritional Info: Calories: 200, Protein: 8g, Fat: 8g, Carbohydrates: 28g

Tofu Stir-Fry

A flavorful stir-fry made with tofu, colorful vegetables, and a tangy ginger-soy sauce.

Preparation Time: 15 minutes, Cooking Time: 15 minutes, Total Time: 30 minutes, serving: 4

Ingredients: 1 block (14 oz) firm tofu, pressed and cubed, 2 cups mixed vegetables (such as bell peppers, broccoli, and snap peas), chopped, 2 cloves garlic, minced, 1 tbsp grated ginger, 2 tbsp soy sauce (or tamari for gluten-free), 1 tbsp maple syrup, 1 tbsp cornstarch, Cooked brown rice for serving

Directions:

1. In a wok or large skillet, stir-fry tofu cubes over medium-high heat until golden brown. Remove stay-fried tofu from the pan and set aside.
2. In the same pan, stir-fry mixed vegetables, garlic, and ginger until vegetables are tender-crisp.
3. In a small bowl, whisk together soy sauce, maple syrup, and cornstarch.
4. Return tofu to the pan and pour the sauce over the tofu and vegetables. Stir well to coat.
5. Cook for another 2-3 minutes until the sauce thickens.
6. Serve hot over cooked brown rice.
Nutritional Info: Calories: 320, Protein: 18g, Fat: 10g, Carbohydrates: 40g

Cauliflower Taco Bowls

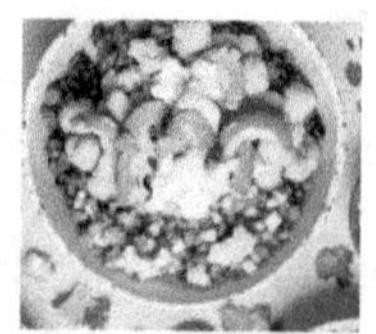

These cauliflower taco bowls are a nutritious and filling option for a protein-packed meal.
Preparation Time: 25 minutes, Cooking Time: 30 minutes, Total Time: 55 minutes, serving: 4
Ingredients: 2 cups cauliflower florets, 1 cup cooked quinoa, 1 cup black beans, 1 cup diced tomatoes, 1/2 cup diced onions, 1/4 cup chopped cilantro, 1 tablespoon lime juice, 1 teaspoon chili powder, 1/2 teaspoon garlic powder.
Direction:
1. Toss cauliflower florets with olive oil, chili powder, and garlic powder. Roast until tender.
2. Assemble bowls with cooked quinoa, roasted cauliflower, black beans, diced tomatoes, diced onions, chopped cilantro, and a squeeze of lime juice.
Nutritional Info: Calories: 230, Protein: 10g, Fat: 6g, Carbohydrates: 32g

Quinoa Stuffed Bell Peppers

Colorful bell peppers stuffed with protein-rich quinoa, black beans, corn, and spices, then baked to perfection.
Preparation Time: 20 minutes, Cooking Time: 30 minutes, Total Time: 50 minutes, serving: 4
Ingredients: 4 bell peppers, halved and seeds removed, 1 cup cooked quinoa, 1 can (15 oz) black beans, drained and rinsed, 1 cup corn kernels (fresh or frozen), 1/2 cup diced tomatoes, 1/4 cup chopped cilantro, 1 tsp chili powder, 1/2 tsp cumin, Juice of 1 lime
Directions:
1. Preheat oven to 375°F (190°C). Place bell pepper halves in a baking dish.
2. In a mixing bowl, combine cooked quinoa, black beans, corn, diced tomatoes, cilantro, chili powder, cumin, and lime juice.
3. Stuff each bell pepper half with the quinoa mixture.
4. Cover the baking dish with aluminum foil and bake until bell peppers are tender, for 25-30 minutes.
5. Serve hot, garnished with additional cilantro if desired.
Nutritional Info: Calories: 270, Protein: 12g, Fat: 2g, Carbohydrates: 50g

Lentil lettuce Tacos

These lentil tacos make a satisfying and protein-packed lunch option.
Meal Time: Lunch, Preparation Time: 20 minutes, Cooking Time: 25 minutes, Total Time: 45 minutes, serving: 4
Ingredients: 8 corn tortillas, 1 cup cooked lentils, 1 cup diced bell peppers, 1 cup diced onions, 1 cup shredded lettuce, 1/2 cup salsa, 1 tablespoon lime juice, 1 teaspoon chili powder, 1/2 teaspoon garlic powder.

Direction:
1. In a skillet, sauté bell peppers and onions until tender.
2. Add cooked lentils, chili powder, and garlic powder, and cook until heated through.
3. Warm corn tortillas and fill each tortilla with lentil mixture, shredded lettuce, salsa, and a squeeze of lime juice.
Nutritional Info: Calories: 200, Protein: 10g, Fat: 5g, Carbohydrates: 30g

Tofu Scramble Tacos

These tofu scramble tacos are a delicious and protein-rich option for any meal.
Meal Time: Anytime, Preparation Time: 20 minutes, Cooking Time: 15 minutes, Total Time: 35 minutes, serving: 4
Ingredients: 8 corn tortillas, 1 block tofu, 1 cup diced bell peppers, 1 cup diced onions, 1/2 cup nutritional yeast, 1/4 cup chopped chives, 1 tablespoon olive oil, 1 teaspoon turmeric, 1/2 teaspoon garlic powder.
Direction:
1. In a skillet, crumble tofu and sauté with olive oil, turmeric, and garlic powder until golden.
2. Add diced bell peppers and onions and cook until softened.
3. Warm corn tortillas. Fill each tortilla with tofu scramble, nutritional yeast, and chopped chives.
Nutritional Info: Calories: 230, Protein: 11g, Fat: 8g, Carbohydrates: 29g

Tofu and Vegetable Quinoa Bowl

This protein-packed quinoa bowl features marinated tofu and a colorful array of vegetables, all served over a bed of fluffy quinoa for a delicious and satisfying lunch.
Preparation Time: 10 minutes, Cooking Time: 15 minutes, Total Time: 25 minutes, Serving Size: 2
Ingredients: 1 cup cooked quinoa, 1 block firm tofu, pressed and cubed, 2 cups mixed vegetables (such as bell peppers, zucchini, mushrooms, and broccoli), 2 cloves garlic, minced, 2 tablespoons low-sodium soy sauce (or tamari for gluten-free), 1 tablespoon rice vinegar, 1 tablespoon maple syrup, 1 teaspoon cornstarch, 2 tablespoons water, Fresh cilantro for garnish
Directions:
1. Cook quinoa according to package instructions and put aside.
2. In a small bowl, whisk together soy sauce, rice vinegar, maple syrup, cornstarch, and water to make the sauce. Set aside.
3. Heat a non-stick skillet over medium heat and add cubed tofu. Cook the cubed tofu for about 5-7 minutes or until golden brown on all sides. Remove the tofu from the heat and set aside.
4. In the same skillet, add minced garlic and mixed vegetables. Cook until tender-crisp, about 5 minutes.
5. Return the tofu to the skillet and pour the sauce over the tofu and vegetables. Cook until the sauce is thickens for another 2minutes or more.
6. Serve hot over cooked quinoa, garnished with fresh cilantro.

Nutritional Info (per serving without quinoa): Calories: 280 Protein: 18g Carbohydrates: 30g Fat: 10g Fiber: 8g

Chickpea Salad with Avocado Dressing

This creamy chickpea salad is dressed with a zesty avocado dressing and served over a bed of mixed greens for a satisfying and nutritious lunch.

Preparation Time: 10 minutes, Cooking Time: 0 minutes, Total Time: 10 minutes, Serving Size: 2

Ingredients: 1 can chickpeas, drained and rinsed, 2 cups mixed greens,1/2 cup cherry tomatoes, halved, 1/4 cup sliced cucumber, 1/4 cup diced red bell pepper, 1/4 cup diced red onion, 2 tablespoons chopped fresh parsley,1 ripe avocado, 2 tablespoons lemon juice, Salt and pepper to taste

Directions:

1. In a large bowl, combine chickpeas, mixed greens, cherry tomatoes, cucumber, red bell pepper, red onion, and fresh parsley.
2. In a blender or food processor, combine ripe avocado, lemon juice, salt, and pepper. Blend until smooth and creamy.
3. Pour the avocado dressing over the salad and toss gently until everything is well coated.
4. Divide into serving bowls and enjoy this creamy and delicious salad!

Nutritional Info (per serving), Calories: 320 Protein: 10g Carbohydrates: 25g Fat: 18g Fiber: 12g

Tempeh Lettuce Wraps

These flavorful lettuce wraps feature marinated tempeh and crisp vegetables, all wrapped in fresh lettuce leaves for a light and satisfying lunch.

Preparation Time: 10 minutes, Cooking Time: 15 minutes, Total Time: 25 minutes, Serving Size: 2

Ingredients: 1 package tempeh, sliced into strips. 1/4 cup low-sodium soy sauce (or tamari for gluten-free), 2 tablespoons rice vinegar, 1 tablespoon maple syrup, 1 clove garlic, minced, 1 teaspoon grated ginger, 1/2 cup shredded carrots, 1/2 cup thinly sliced cucumber, 1/4 cup chopped fresh cilantro, 1/4 cup chopped roasted peanuts (optional), 8 large lettuce leaves (such as butter or romaine)

Directions:

1. In a shallow dish, whisk together soy sauce, rice vinegar, maple syrup, minced garlic, and grated ginger to make the marinade.
2. Add sliced tempeh to the marinade, making sure to coat each piece evenly, set aside to marinate for at least 10 minutes.
3. Heat a non-stick skillet over medium heat and add marinated tempeh slices. Cook until golden brown on both sides, about 3 minutes per side.
4. In a bowl, combine shredded carrots, sliced cucumber, chopped cilantro, and chopped roasted peanuts (if using).
5. To assemble the lettuce wraps, place a spoonful of the vegetable mixture and a few slices of cooked tempeh onto each lettuce leaf.
6. Roll up the lettuce leaves, enclosing the filling, and secure with toothpicks if needed.
7. Serve immediately and enjoy these delicious and nutritious tempeh lettuce wraps!

Nutritional Info (per serving): Calories: 280 Protein: 15g Carbohydrates: 20g Fat: 14g Fiber: 8g

Tofu and Vegetable Buddha Bowl

This nourishing Buddha bowl features marinated tofu, roasted vegetables, and a tangy tahini dressing for a hearty and flavorful lunch.

Preparation Time: 10 minutes, Cooking Time: 25 minutes, Total Time: 35 minutes, Serving Size: 2

Ingredients: 1 block firm tofu, pressed and cubed, 2 cups mixed vegetables (such as sweet potatoes, Brussels sprouts, and cauliflower), 2 tablespoons low-sodium soy sauce (or tamari for gluten-free), 1 tablespoon rice vinegar, 1 tablespoon maple syrup, 1 teaspoon sesame oil (optional, omit for oil-free)1/4 cup tahini, 2 tablespoons lemon juice, 1 clove garlic, minced, Cooked quinoa or brown rice for serving

Directions:

1. Preheat the oven to 400°F (200°C) and line a baking sheet with parchment paper.
2. In a shallow dish, whisk together soy sauce, rice vinegar, maple syrup, and sesame oil (if using) to make the marinade.
3. Add cubed tofu to the marinade, making sure to coat each piece evenly. Let it marinate for at least 10 minutes or more.
4. Place marinated tofu on one half of the prepared baking sheet.
5. On the other half of the baking sheet, arrange mixed vegetables in a single layer.
6. Roast in the preheated oven for 20-25 minutes, flipping tofu halfway through, until tofu is golden brown and vegetables are tender.
7. In a small bowl, whisk together tahini, lemon juice, minced garlic, and water to make the dressing.
8. To assemble the Buddha bowls, divide cooked quinoa or brown rice between serving bowls.
9. Top with roasted tofu and vegetables, and drizzle with tahini dressing.
10. Serve immediately and enjoy this delicious and wholesome Buddha bowl!

Nutritional Info (per serving without rice/quinoa): Calories: 320 Protein: 16g Carbohydrates: 30g Fat: 18g, Fiber: 8g

Mediterranean Chickpea Salad

This vibrant salad features protein-packed chickpeas, crisp vegetables, and tangy olives, all tossed in a zesty lemon-herb dressing for a refreshing and satisfying lunch.

Preparation Time: 15 minutes, Cooking Time: 0 minutes, Total Time: 15 minutes, Serving Size: 2

Ingredients:1 can chickpeas, drained and rinsed, 1 cup cherry tomatoes, halved, 1/2 cucumber, diced, 1/4 cup diced red onion, 1/4 cup sliced Kalamata olives, 2 tablespoons chopped fresh parsley,2 tablespoons lemon juice, 1 tablespoon olive oil (optional, omit for oil-free), 1 teaspoon dried oregano, Salt and pepper to taste

Directions:

1. In a large bowl, combine chickpeas, cucumber, cherry tomatoes, Kalamata olives, red onion, and fresh parsley.

2. In a small bowl, whisk together lemon juice, olive oil (if using), dried oregano, salt, and pepper to make the dressing.

3. Pour the dressing over the salad and toss gently until everything is well coated.

4. Divide into serving bowls and enjoy this flavorful and nutritious Mediterranean chickpea salad!

Nutritional Info (per serving): Calories: 290 Protein: 10g Carbohydrates: 30g Fat: 14g Fiber: 10g

Lentil and Vegetable Soup

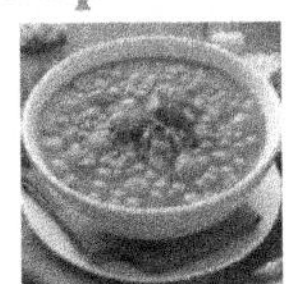

This hearty soup features protein-rich lentils, flavorful vegetables, and aromatic spices for a comforting and nutritious lunch.

Preparation Time: 10 minutes, Cooking Time: 25 minutes, Total Time: 35 minutes, Serving Size: 2

Ingredients: 1 cup cooked lentils, 2 cups vegetable broth 1 cup diced tomatoes,1/2 cup diced carrots, 1/2 cup diced celery, 1/4 cup diced onion,2 cloves garlic, minced,1 teaspoon ground cumin, 1/2 teaspoon smoked paprika, Salt and pepper to taste, Fresh parsley for garnish

Directions:

1. In a large pot, combine cooked lentils, vegetable broth, diced tomatoes, carrots, celery, onion, minced garlic, ground cumin, and smoked paprika.

2. Increase the heat to medium-high heat and it boil.

3. Reduce heat to low, cover, and simmer for 20-25 minutes until vegetables are tender.

4. Season with salt and pepper to taste.

5. Ladle the soup into serving bowls, garnish with fresh parsley, and serve hot.

Nutritional Info (per serving): Calories: 250 Protein: 15g Carbohydrates: 35g Fat: 2g Fiber: 12g

Stuffed Bell Peppers with Quinoa and Beans

These colorful bell peppers are stuffed with protein-rich quinoa, black beans, and vegetables, making them a delicious and nutritious lunch option.

Preparation Time: 15 minutes Cooking Time: 30 minutes Total Time: 45 minutes Serving Size: 2

Ingredients: 2 large bell peppers, any color, 1 cup cooked quinoa, 1/2 cup black beans, drained and rinsed, 1/2 cup corn kernels (fresh or frozen), 1/4 cup diced tomatoes, 1/4 cup diced red onion, 2 cloves garlic, minced, 1 teaspoon ground cumin, 1/2 teaspoon chili powder, Salt and pepper to taste, Fresh cilantro for garnish

Directions:

1. Preheat the oven to 375°F (190°C) and line a baking dish with parchment paper.

2. Properly cut the tops off the bell peppers and remove the seeds and membranes.

3. In a large bowl, mix together cooked quinoa, black beans, corn kernels, diced tomatoes, red onion, minced garlic, ground cumin, chili powder, salt, and pepper.
4. Stuff each bell pepper with the quinoa and bean mixture, pressing down gently to pack it in.
5. Place the stuffed bell peppers in the prepared baking dish and cover with foil.
6. Bake for 25-30 minutes until the peppers are tender.
7. Remove from the oven, garnish with fresh cilantro, and serve hot.
Nutritional Info (per serving): Calories: 300 Protein: 12g Carbohydrates: 50g Fat: 3g Fiber: 10g

DINNER RECIPES

These recipes offer a variety of delicious and nutritious options for a high-protein plant-based dinner without oil salt. Enjoy experimenting with these flavors and ingredients!

Lentil and Vegetable Curry

A hearty and flavorful curry made with protein-rich lentils, assorted vegetables, and aromatic spices, perfect for a comforting dinner.

Preparation Time: 15 minutes, Cooking Time: 30 minutes. Total Time: 45 minutes, Serving Size: 4

Ingredients: 1 cup dry lentils, 2 cups vegetable broth, 1 onion, diced, 2 cloves garlic, minced, 1 tablespoon curry powder, 1 teaspoon ground cumin, 1 teaspoon ground turmeric, 1 can diced tomatoes, 2 cups chopped mixed vegetables (such as carrots, bell peppers, and cauliflower), 1 cup coconut milk, Fresh cilantro for garnish

Directions:
1. Rinse lentils thoroughly and drain.
2. In a large pot, combine lentils, vegetable broth, diced onion, minced garlic, curry powder, cumin, turmeric, diced tomatoes, and mixed vegetables.
3. Bring to a boil, then reduce heat and simmer for 25-30 minutes until lentils are tender and vegetables are cooked.
4. Stir in coconut milk and simmer for an additional 5 minutes.
5. Garnish with fresh cilantro before serving. Enjoy with rice or naan bread.
Nutritional Info (per serving): Calories: 350 Protein: 15g Carbohydrates: 50g Fat: 10g Fiber: 12g

Chickpea and Vegetable Stir-Fry

A quick and easy stir-fry featuring protein-packed chickpeas, colorful vegetables, and savory seasonings, perfect for a nutritious dinner.

Preparation Time: 15 minutes, Cooking Time: 15 minutes, Total Time: 30 minutes, Serving Size: 4

Ingredients: 2 cans chickpeas, drained and rinsed, 2 cups mixed vegetables (such as bell peppers, broccoli, and snap peas), 1 onion, sliced, 2 cloves garlic, minced, 2 tablespoons low-sodium soy sauce (or tamari for gluten-free), 1 tablespoon rice vinegar, 1 tablespoon maple syrup, 1 teaspoon cornstarch, 2 tablespoons water
Directions:
1. In a small bowl, whisk together soy sauce, rice vinegar, maple syrup, cornstarch, and water to make the sauce. Set aside.
2. Heat a large skillet over medium heat and add sliced onion and minced garlic. Cook until softened, about 2-3 minutes.
3. Add mixed vegetables to the skillet and cook until tender-crisp, about 5 minutes.
4. Stir in chickpeas and sauce mixture. Cook for an additional 3-4 minutes until heated through and sauce has thickened.
5. Serve hot over cooked quinoa or brown rice.
Nutritional Info (per serving without rice/quinoa): Calories: 300 Protein: 14g Carbohydrates: 40g Fat: 8g Fiber: 10g

Quinoa and Black Bean Stuffed Bell Peppers

Colorful bell peppers stuffed with protein-rich quinoa, black beans, and vegetables, baked to perfection for a wholesome and satisfying dinner.
Preparation Time: 15 minutes, Cooking Time: 30 minutes, Total Time: 45 minutes, Serving Size: 4
Ingredients: 4 large bell peppers, any color, 1 cup cooked quinoa, 1 can black beans, drained and rinsed, 1 cup corn kernels (fresh or frozen), 1/2 cup diced tomatoes, 1/4 cup diced red onion, 2 cloves garlic, minced, 1 teaspoon cumin, 1/2 teaspoon chili powder, Fresh cilantro for garnish
Directions:
1. Preheat the oven to 375°F (190°C) and line a baking dish with parchment paper.
2. Cut the tops off the bell peppers and remove the seeds and membranes.
3. In a large bowl, mix together cooked quinoa, black beans, corn kernels, diced tomatoes, red onion, minced garlic, cumin, and chili powder.
4. Stuff each bell pepper with the quinoa and black bean mixture, pressing down gently to pack it in.
5. Place the stuffed bell peppers in the prepared baking dish and cover with foil.
6. Bake for 25-30 minutes until the peppers are tender.
7. Remove from the oven, garnish with fresh cilantro, and serve hot.
Nutritional Info (per serving): Calories: 320 Protein: 15g Carbohydrates: 45g Fat: 3g Fiber: 10g

Mushroom Walnut Tacos

These tacos are a delicious dinner option, filled with savory mushrooms and crunchy walnuts.
Preparation Time: 20 minutes, Cooking Time: 15 minutes, Total Time: 35 minutes, serving: 4
Ingredients: 8 corn tortillas, 2 cups sliced mushrooms, 1 cup chopped walnuts, 1/4 cup diced onions, 1/4 cup chopped cilantro, 2 tablespoons lime juice, 1 teaspoon cumin, 1 teaspoon smoked paprika, 1/2 teaspoon garlic powder.
Direction:

1. In a skillet, sauté mushrooms and onions until tender.
2. Add chopped walnuts and spices, cook until fragrant.
3. Warm tortillas and fill with mushroom-walnut mixture.
4. Top with chopped cilantro and a squeeze of lime juice and Serve hot.
Nutritional Info: Calories: 210, Protein: 9g, Fat: 10g, Carbohydrates: 25g

BBQ Jackfruit Tacos

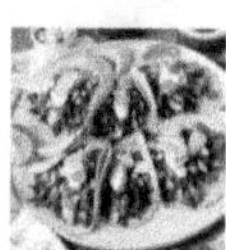

These BBQ jackfruit tacos are a flavorful and satisfying option for a protein-rich meal.
Preparation Time: 25 minutes, Cooking Time: 30 minutes, Total Time: 55 minutes, serving: 4
Ingredients: 8 corn tortillas, 2 cups shredded jackfruit, 1 cup diced onions, 1 cup diced bell peppers, 1/2 cup BBQ sauce, 1/4 cup chopped cilantro, 1 tablespoon olive oil, 1 teaspoon garlic powder, 1/2 teaspoon smoked paprika.
Direction:
1. In a skillet, sauté onions and bell peppers with olive oil, garlic powder, and smoked paprika until tender.
2. Add shredded jackfruit and BBQ sauce, and cook until heated through.
3. Warm corn tortillas and fill each tortilla with BBQ jackfruit mixture and chopped cilantro.
Nutritional Info: Calories: 230, Protein: 8g, Fat: 8g, Carbohydrates: 32g

Sweet Potato Tacos

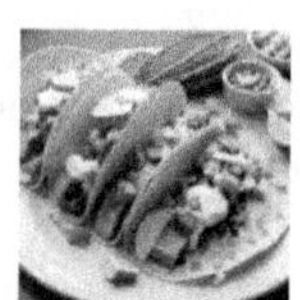

These sweet potato tacos are a delicious and nutritious option for a satisfying meal.
Preparation Time: 20 minutes, Cooking Time: 25 minutes, Total Time: 45 minutes, serving: 4
Ingredients: 8 corn tortillas, 2 cups diced sweet potatoes, 1 cup black beans, 1 cup diced tomatoes, 1/2 cup diced onions, 1/4 cup chopped cilantro, 1 tablespoon olive oil, 1 teaspoon chili powder, 1/2 teaspoon cumin.
Direction:
1. Toss sweet potatoes with olive oil, chili powder, and cumin. Roast until tender.
2. Warm corn tortillas and Fill each tortilla with roasted sweet potatoes, black beans, diced tomatoes, diced onions, and chopped cilantro.
Nutritional Info: Calories: 220, Protein: 9g, Fat: 7g, Carbohydrates: 30g

Greek Chickpea Tacos

These Greek chickpea tacos are a flavorful and protein-packed option for a quick and easy meal.
Meal Time: Anytime, Preparation Time: 15 minutes, Cooking Time: 10 minutes,
Total Time: 25 minutes, serving: 4
Ingredients: 8 corn tortillas, 2 cups cooked chickpeas, 1 cup diced cucumbers, 1
cup diced tomatoes, 1/2 cup diced red onions, 1/4 cup chopped Kalamata olives,
1/4 cup chopped parsley, 1 tablespoon lemon juice, 1 tablespoon olive oil, 1
teaspoon dried oregano.
Direction:
1. In a bowl, combine cooked chickpeas, diced cucumbers, diced tomatoes, diced
red onions, chopped Kalamata olives, parsley, lemon juice, olive oil, and dried
oregano. Mix well.
2. Warm corn tortillas and Fill each tortilla with the chickpea mixture. Enjoy!
Nutritional Info: Calories: 240, Protein: 9g, Fat: 7g, Carbohydrates: 32g

Spicy Chickpea Tacos

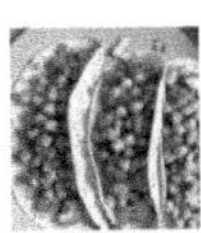

These spicy chickpea tacos are a flavorful option for a quick and satisfying dinner.
Preparation Time: 15 minutes, Cooking Time: 20 minutes, Total Time: 35 minutes
Serving: 4
Ingredients: 8 corn tortillas, 2 cups cooked chickpeas, 1 cup diced tomatoes, 1 cup
diced onions, 1/2 cup chopped cilantro, 1/4 cup hot sauce, 1 tablespoon lime juice,
1 teaspoon chili powder, 1/2 teaspoon garlic powder.
Direction:
1. In a skillet, sauté cooked chickpeas with diced tomatoes, onions, chili powder,
and garlic powder until heated through.
2. Warm corn tortillas and fill each tortilla with chickpea mixture, chopped cilantro,
hot sauce, and a squeeze of lime juice.
Nutritional Info: Calories: 210, Protein: 9g, Fat: 6g, Carbohydrates: 32g

Chickpea and Vegetable Quinoa Bowl

A satisfying bowl filled with protein-packed chickpeas, colorful vegetables, and fluffy quinoa.
**Preparation Time: 10 minutes, Cooking Time: 20 minutes, Total Time: 30
minutes serving: 4**
Ingredients:1 cup quinoa, 1 can chickpeas, drained and rinsed, 1 cup diced bell
peppers, 1 cup diced cucumber, 1 cup cherry tomatoes, halved, 1/2 cup diced red
onion, 2 tablespoons chopped parsleyJuice of 1 lemon
Directions:
1. Cook quinoa according to package instructions.
2. In a bowl, combine cooked quinoa, chickpeas, bell peppers, cucumber, cherry
tomatoes, red onion, and parsley.
3. Squeeze lemon juice over the bowl and toss to combine. Serve and enjoy!
Nutritional Info: Calories: 250, Protein: 11g, Fat: 3g, Carbohydrates: 45g

Quinoa and Edamame Salad

Refreshing salad featuring protein-packed quinoa, edamame, and crunchy vegetables.
Preparation Time: 15 minutes, Cooking Time: 15 minutes, Total Time: 30 minutes, serving: 4
Ingredients: 1 cup quinoa, 1 cup shelled edamame, thawed if frozen, 1 cup diced cucumber, 1 cup diced bell peppers, 1/2 cup shredded carrots, 2 tablespoons chopped fresh ,1/4 cup chopped green onions, cilantro, Juice of 2 limes
Directions:
1. Cook quinoa according to package instructions.
2. In a large bowl, combine cooked quinoa, edamame, cucumber, bell peppers, carrots, green onions, cilantro, and lime juice.
3. Toss until well mixed. Enjoy!
Nutritional Info: Calories: 240, Protein: 12g, Fat: 4g, Carbohydrates: 40g

Tofu and Vegetable Stir-Fry

A flavorful stir-fry featuring marinated tofu and crisp vegetables, all tossed in a savory sauce for a delicious and satisfying dinner.
Preparation Time: 15 minutes, Cooking Time: 15 minutes, Total Time: 30 minutes, Serving Size: 4
Ingredients: 1 block firm tofu, pressed and cubed, 2 cups mixed vegetables (such as bell peppers, broccoli, and snap peas), 2 cloves garlic, minced, 2 tablespoons low-sodium soy sauce (or tamari for gluten-free), 1 tablespoon rice vinegar, 1 tablespoon maple syrup, 1 teaspoon cornstarch, 2 tablespoons water
Directions:
1. In a small bowl, whisk together soy sauce, rice vinegar, maple syrup, cornstarch, and water to make the sauce. Set aside.
2. Heat a large skillet over medium heat and add cubed tofu. Cook for about 6-7 minutes or until golden brown on all sides. Remove tofu from the skillet and set aside.
3. In the same skillet, add minced garlic and mixed vegetables. Cook until tender-crisp, about 5 minutes.
4. Return the tofu to the skillet and pour the sauce over the tofu and vegetables. Cook for more 2-3 minutes until the sauce thickens.
5. Serve hot over cooked quinoa or brown rice.
Nutritional Info (per serving without rice/quinoa): Calories: 280, Protein: 16g, Carbohydrates: 30g, Fat: 10g, Fiber: 8g

Chili Sin Carne

A hearty and flavorful chili made with protein-packed beans, vegetables, and spices, perfect for a comforting and satisfying dinner.
Preparation Time: 15 minutes, Cooking Time: 30 minutes, Total Time: 45 minutes Serving: 4
Ingredients: 1 can black beans, drained and rinsed, 1 can kidney beans, drained and rinsed, 1 can diced tomatoes, 1 onion, diced, 2 cloves garlic, minced, 1 bell pepper, diced, 1 teaspoon ground cumin, 1 cup corn kernels (fresh or frozen), 2

tablespoons tomato paste, 1 tablespoon chili powder, 1 teaspoon smoked paprika, Salt and pepper to taste

Directions:

1. In a large pot, sauté diced onion, minced garlic, and diced bell pepper until softened, about 2-3 minutes.
2. Add black beans, kidney beans, diced tomatoes, corn kernels, tomato paste, chili powder, cumin, smoked paprika, salt, and pepper to the pot.
3. Stir well to combine and bring to a simmer.
4. Cook for 20-25 minutes, stirring occasionally, until flavors are well blended and chili has thickened.
5. Serve hot, garnished with fresh cilantro or sliced green onions.

Nutritional Info (per serving): Calories: 300, Protein: 15g, Carbohydrates: 45g, Fat: 2g, Fiber: 12g

Stuffed Portobello Mushrooms with Quinoa and Spinach

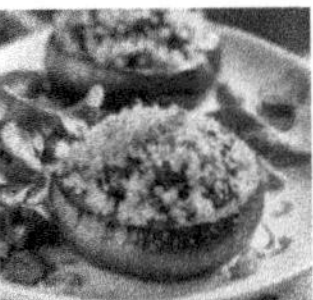

These hearty portobello mushrooms are stuffed with protein-rich quinoa, flavorful spinach, and aromatic herbs.

Preparation Time: 15 minutes, Cooking Time: 25 minutes, Total Time: 40 minutes, serving: 4

Ingredients: 4 large portobello mushrooms, 1 cup cooked quinoa, 2 cups chopped spinach, 1/4 cup diced onion, 2 cloves garlic, minced, 1 teaspoon dried oregano, 2 tablespoons nutritional yeast, 1 teaspoon dried thyme, Salt and pepper to taste, Fresh parsley for garnish

Directions:

1. Preheat the oven to 375°F (190°C) and line a baking sheet with parchment paper.
2. Remove the stems from the portobello mushrooms and gently scrape out the gills using a spoon.
3. In a medium skillet, sauté diced onion and minced garlic until softened, for about 2-3 minutes.
4. Add chopped spinach to the skillet and cook until wilted, about 2 minutes.
5. In a large bowl, mix together cooked quinoa, sautéed spinach mixture, nutritional yeast, dried thyme, dried oregano, salt, and pepper.
6. Divide the quinoa mixture evenly among the portobello mushrooms, pressing down gently to pack it in.
7. Place the stuffed mushrooms on the prepared baking sheet and bake for 20-25 minutes until mushrooms are tender.
8. Remove from the oven, garnish with fresh parsley, and serve hot.

Nutritional Info (per serving): Calories: 250, Protein: 12g, Carbohydrates: 30g, Fat: 5g, Fiber: 8g

Chickpea and Spinach Coconut Curry

A creamy and aromatic coconut curry featuring protein-packed chickpeas, tender spinach, and fragrant spices, perfect for a cozy dinner.

Preparation Time: 15 minutes, Cooking Time: 25 minutes, Total Time: 40 minutes, Serving Size: 4

Ingredients: 2 cans chickpeas, drained and rinsed, 2 cups chopped spinach, 1 onion, diced, 2 cloves garlic, minced, 1 tablespoon curry powder, 1 teaspoon ground turmeric, 1 can coconut milk, 1 cup vegetable broth, 1 tablespoon coconut oil (optional, omit for oil-free), Fresh cilantro for garnish

Directions:

1. In a large pot, sauté diced onion and minced garlic in coconut oil (if using) until softened, about 2-3 minutes.

2. Add curry powder and ground turmeric to the pot and cook until fragrant. For another 1-2 minutes.

3. Stir in chickpeas, chopped spinach, coconut milk, and vegetable broth.

4. Bring to a simmer and cook for 20-25 minutes until flavors are well blended and curry has thickened.

5. Serve hot, garnished with fresh cilantro, and enjoy with rice or naan bread.

Nutritional Info (per serving): Calories: 320 Protein: 14g Carbohydrates: 40g Fat: 12g Fiber: 10g

Tofu and Vegetable Sheet Pan Dinner

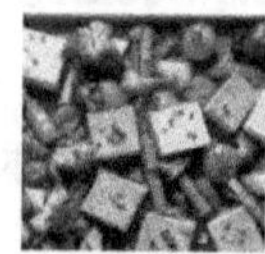

An easy and versatile sheet pan dinner featuring marinated tofu, roasted vegetables, and aromatic herbs, perfect for a hassle-free dinner.

Preparation Time: 15 minutes, Cooking Time: 25 minutes. Total Time: 40 minutes, serving: 4

Ingredients: 1 block firm tofu, pressed and cubed, 4 cups mixed vegetables (such as bell peppers, broccoli, carrots, and cauliflower), 2 tablespoons balsamic vinegar, 1 tablespoon Dijon mustard, 1 tablespoon maple syrup, 2 cloves garlic, minced, 1 teaspoon dried thyme, 1 teaspoon dried rosemary, Fresh parsley for garnish

Directions:

1. Preheat the oven to 400°F (200°C) and line a baking sheet with parchment paper.

2. In a small bowl, whisk together balsamic vinegar, Dijon mustard, maple syrup, minced garlic, dried thyme, and dried rosemary to make the marinade.

3. Place cubed tofu and mixed vegetables on the prepared baking sheet.

4. Drizzle marinade over tofu and vegetables, tossing to coat evenly.

5. Spread tofu and vegetables out in a single layer on the baking sheet.

6. Bake for 20-25 minutes until tofu is golden brown and vegetables are tender.

7. Serve hot, garnished with fresh parsley.

Nutritional Info (per serving): Calories: 280, Protein: 16g, Carbohydrates: 30g, Fat: 10g Fiber: 8g

Mushroom and Lentil Shepherd's Pie

A hearty and comforting shepherd's pie featuring savory mushrooms, protein-rich lentils, and creamy mashed potatoes, perfect for a cozy dinner.

Preparation Time: 20 minutes, Cooking Time: 40 minutes, Total Time: 1 hour, Serving Size: 4

Ingredients: 2 cups cooked lentils, 2 cups sliced mushrooms, 1 onion, diced, 2 cloves garlic, minced, 1 cup frozen peas, 2 tablespoons tomato paste, 1 teaspoon dried thyme, 1 teaspoon dried rosemary, 4 cups mashed potatoes (made without dairy), Fresh parsley for garnish

Directions:

1. Preheat the oven to 375°F (190°C).
2. In a large skillet, sauté diced onion and minced garlic until softened, about 2-3 minutes.
3. Add sliced mushrooms to the skillet and cook until browned, about 5 minutes.
4. Stir in cooked lentils, frozen peas, tomato paste, dried thyme, and dried rosemary. Cook for another 2-3 minutes until heated through.
5. Transfer the mushroom and lentil mixture to a baking dish and spread mashed potatoes evenly over the top.
6. Bake for 25-30 minutes until the edges are bubbly and the mashed potatoes are golden brown.
7. Serve hot, garnished with fresh parsley.

Nutritional Info (per serving): Calories: 320, Protein: 14g, Carbohydrates: 45g, Fat: 8g, Fiber: 12g

Eggplant and Chickpea Tagine

A fragrant and flavorful Moroccan-inspired tagine featuring tender eggplant, protein-packed chickpeas, and aromatic spices, perfect for a unique and satisfying dinner.

Preparation Time: 20 minutes, Cooking Time: 40 minutes, Total Time: 1 hour, serving: 4

Ingredients: 1 large eggplant, diced, 1 can chickpeas, drained and rinsed, 1 onion, diced, 2 cloves garlic, minced, 1 teaspoon ground cumin, 1 teaspoon ground coriander, 1/2 teaspoon ground cinnamon, 1/4 teaspoon cayenne pepper, 1 can diced tomatoes, 1 cup vegetable broth, 1/4 cup chopped dried apricots, 2 tablespoons chopped fresh parsley, Cooked couscous for serving

Directions:

1. In a large pot or Dutch oven, sauté diced onion and minced garlic until softened, about 2-3 minutes.
2. Add diced eggplant to the pot and cook until softened, about 5 minutes.

3. Stir in ground cumin, ground coriander, ground cinnamon, and cayenne pepper. Cook for more few minutes or until fragrant.
4. Add chickpeas, diced tomatoes, vegetable broth, and chopped dried apricots to the pot. Stir well to combine.
5. Bring to a simmer and cook for 25-30 minutes until flavors are well blended and tagine has thickened.
6. Serve hot, garnished with chopped fresh parsley, and enjoy with cooked couscous.
Nutritional Info (per serving without couscous): Calories: 280 Protein: 12g Carbohydrates: 40g Fat: 8g Fiber: 10g

DESSERT RECIPES

These dessert recipes offer a delightful array of flavors and textures, perfect for satisfying your sweet tooth while maintaining a healthy, plant-based lifestyle. Enjoy experimenting with these delicious treats!

Chocolate Avocado Mousse

Creamy and decadent chocolate mousse made with ripe avocados and cocoa powder, perfect for a guilt-free indulgence.

Preparation Time: 10 minutes, Cooking Time: 0 minutes, Total Time: 10 minutes, serving: 2

Ingredients: 2 ripe avocados, 1/4 cup cocoa powder, 1/4 cup maple syrup or agave nectar, 1 teaspoon vanilla extract, Fresh berries for garnish

Directions:
1. Scoop the flesh of the avocados into a bowl of a blender or food processor.
2. Add cocoa powder, maple syrup or agave nectar, and vanilla extract.
3. Blend the mixture until smooth and creamy, scraping down the sides of the blender bowl or food processor bowl as needed.
4. Divide into serving bowls, garnish with fresh berries, and refrigerate for 1 hour before serving.

Nutritional Info (per serving): Calories: 300, Protein: 5g, Carbohydrates: 25g, Fat: 20g, Fiber: 10g

Peanut Butter Banana Protein Bites

Chewy and satisfying bites made with mashed bananas, peanut butter, and protein powder, perfect for a quick and energizing snack.

Preparation Time: 10 minutes, Cooking Time: 0 minutes, Total Time: 10 minutes, serving: 4

Ingredients: 2 ripe bananas, mashed, 1/4 cup peanut butter, 1/4 cup protein powder (vanilla or chocolate flavored), 1/4 cup rolled oats, 1 tablespoon chia seeds (optional)

Directions:

1. In a mixing bowl, combine mashed bananas, peanut butter, protein powder, rolled oats, and chia seeds (if using).

2. Mix until well combined and a dough forms.

3. Roll the dough into bite-sized balls using your hands.

4. Place the balls on a baking sheet lined with parchment paper and refrigerate for about30 minutes before serving.

Nutritional Info (per serving):. Calories: 200, Protein: 10g, Carbohydrates: 20g, Fat: 8g, Fiber: 5g

Chia Seed Pudding

A creamy and nutritious pudding made with chia seeds and almond milk, flavored with vanilla and sweetened with maple syrup.

Preparation Time: 5 minutes, Cooking Time: 0 minutes, Total Time: 5 minutes (plus chilling time), serving: 2

Ingredients: 1/4 cup chia seeds, 1 cup almond milk, 1 tablespoon maple syrup, 1/2 teaspoon vanilla, extract. Fresh fruit for topping

Directions:

1. In a mixing bowl, whisk together chia seeds, almond milk, maple syrup, and vanilla extract.

2. Let the mixture sit for 5 minutes, then whisk again to break up any clumps.

3. Cover the bowl and refrigerate for at least 2 hours or overnight until thickened.

4. Serve chilled, topped with fresh fruit of your choice.

Nutritional Info (per serving): Calories: 150, Protein: 5g, Carbohydrates: 15g, Fat: 8g, Fiber: 10g

Baked Apples with Cinnamon and Almonds

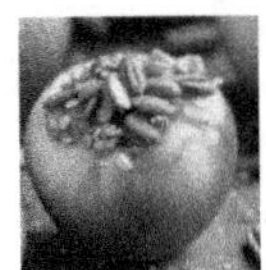

Tender baked apples filled with cinnamon-spiced almonds, a simple and comforting dessert that's perfect for any occasion.

Preparation Time: 10 minutes, Cooking Time: 30 minutes, Total Time: 40 minutes, serving: 2

Ingredients: 2 apples, cored, 1/4 cup chopped almonds, 1 tablespoon maple syrup, 1 teaspoon cinnamon 1/4 teaspoon nutmeg, 1/4 teaspoon vanilla extract, Coconut yogurt for serving (optional)

Directions:

1. Preheat the oven to 375°F (190°C) and line a baking dish with parchment paper.

2. In a small bowl, combine chopped almonds, maple syrup, cinnamon, nutmeg, and vanilla extract.

3. Stuff each cored apple with the almond mixture.

4. Place the stuffed apples in the prepared baking dish and cover with foil.
5. Bake for 25-30 minutes until apples are tender.
6. Serve hot, optionally topped with coconut yogurt.
Nutritional Info (per serving): Calories: 250 Protein: 5g Carbohydrates: 30g Fat: 12g Fiber: 8g

Banana Oatmeal Cookies

Soft and chewy cookies made with mashed bananas, oats, and a hint of cinnamon, perfect for a wholesome and satisfying treat.

Preparation Time: 10 minutes, Cooking Time: 15 minutes, Total Time: 25 minutes, serving: 4

Ingredients: 2 ripe bananas, mashed, 1 cup rolled oats, 1/4 cup chopped nuts (such as almonds or walnuts), 1/4 cup raisins or dried cranberries, 1 teaspoon cinnamon, 1/2 teaspoon vanilla extract

Directions:

1. Preheat the oven to 350°F (175°C) and line a baking sheet with parchment paper.
2. In a mixing bowl, combine mashed bananas, rolled oats, chopped nuts, raisins or dried cranberries, cinnamon, and vanilla extract.
3. Mix until well combined.
4. Drop spoonfuls of the dough onto the prepared baking sheet and flatten slightly with the back of a spoon.
5. Bake for 12-15 minutes until cookies are golden brown.
6. Allow to cool before serving.

Nutritional Info (per serving): Calories: 200 Protein: 5g Carbohydrates: 25g Fat: 8g Fiber: 5g

Chocolate Protein Balls

Decadent chocolate protein balls packed with plant-based protein and natural sweetness.

Preparation Time: 10 minutes,Cooking Time: 0 minutes, Total Time: 10 minutes,serving: 12

Ingredients: 1 cup rolled oats, 1/2 cup almond butter,1/4 cup maple syrup, 2 tablespoons cocoa powder, 2 tablespoons vegan chocolate protein powder, 1/4 cup chopped nuts (such as almonds or walnuts)

Directions:

1. In a mixing bowl, combine rolled oats, maple syrup, cocoa powder, almond butter, vegan chocolate chopped nuts and protein powder. Mix until well combined.
2. Roll the mixture into small balls.
3. Place in the refrigerator to firm up before serving.

Nutritional Info: Calories: 150, Protein: 6g, Fat: 7g, Carbohydrates: 18g

Peanut Butter Banana Nice Cream

Creamy and indulgent nice cream made with frozen bananas and peanut butter.

Preparation Time: 5 minutes, Cooking Time: 0 minutes, Total Time: 5 minutes, serving: 2

Ingredients: 2 ripe bananas, sliced and frozen, 2 tablespoons peanut butter, 1/4 cup unsweetened almond milk

Directions:

1. In a blender or food processor, blend frozen banana slices, peanut butter, and almond milk until smooth and creamy.

2. Remove from food processor and serve immediately as soft-serve ice cream or transfer to a container and freeze for a firmer texture.

Nutritional Info: Calories: 180, Protein: 5g, Fat: 9g, Carbohydrates: 23g

Vanilla Chia Pudding

Silky vanilla chia pudding sweetened with natural ingredients and packed with protein.

Preparation Time: 5 minutes. Cooking Time: 0 minutes, Total Time: 5 minutes (plus chilling time), serving: 2

Ingredients: 1 tablespoon maple syrup, 1/4 cup chia seeds, 1 cup unsweetened almond milk, 1 teaspoon vanilla extract

Directions:

1. In a mixing bowl, whisk together chia seeds, almond milk, maple syrup, and vanilla extract.

2. Let the mixture sit for 5 minutes, then whisk again to prevent clumping.

3. Cover and refrigerate for at least 2 hours or overnight until thickened.

4. Serve chilled.

Nutritional Info: Calories: 120, Protein: 5g, Fat: 6g, Carbohydrates: 14g

Berry Protein Smoothie Bowl

Refreshing smoothie bowl packed with mixed berries and protein-rich ingredients.

Preparation Time: 5 minutes, Cooking Time: 0 minutes, Total Time: 5 minutes, serving: 1

Ingredients: 1 cup mixed berries (such as strawberries, blueberries, raspberries), 1/2 cup silken tofu, 1/4 cup unsweetened almond milk, 1 tablespoon almond butter, 1 tablespoon chia seeds

Directions:

1. In a blender, combine mixed berries, silken tofu, almond milk, and almond butter. Blend until smooth and creamy.

2. Pour the smoothie into a bowl and top with chia seeds and enjoy!

Nutritional Info: Calories: 220, Protein: 10g, Fat: 10g, Carbohydrates: 25g

Protein-Rich Chocolate Avocado Mousse

Creamy and rich chocolate avocado mousse infused with plant-based protein.

Preparation Time: 10 minutes, Cooking Time: 0 minutes, Total Time: 10 minutes, serving: 4

Ingredients: 2 ripe avocados, 1/4 cup cocoa powder, 1/4 cup maple syrup, 1/4 cup unsweetened almond milk, 2 tablespoons vegan chocolate protein powder
Directions:
1. In a food processor, combine ripe avocados, cocoa powder, maple syrup, almond milk, and vegan chocolate protein powder.
2. Blend until smooth and creamy.
3. Divide into serving cups and chill in the refrigerator before serving.
Nutritional Info: Calories: 220, Protein: 8g, Fat: 14g, Carbohydrates: 22g

Coconut Date Energy Balls

Chewy and flavorful energy balls made with dates, coconut, and almonds, perfect for a quick and nutritious snack on the go.
Preparation Time: 15 minutes, Cooking Time: 0 minutes, Total Time: 15 minutes, serving: 4
Ingredients: 1 cup pitted dates, 1/2 cup shredded coconut 1/4 cup almonds, 1 tablespoon cocoa powder, 1 teaspoon vanilla extract, Pinch of cinnamon
Directions:
1. In a food processor, combine pitted dates, shredded coconut, almonds, cocoa powder, vanilla extract, and cinnamon.
2. Pulse until the mixture forms a sticky dough.
3. Roll the dough into small balls using your hands.
4. Optional: Roll the balls in additional shredded coconut for coating.
5. Refrigerate for 30 minutes before serving.
Nutritional Info (per serving): Calories: 200, Protein: 4g, Carbohydrates: 30g, Fat: 8g, Fiber: 6g

Berry Chia Jam

A simple and naturally sweetened jam made with mixed berries and chia seeds, perfect for spreading on toast or serving with yogurt.
Preparation Time: 5 minutes, Cooking Time: 10 minutes, Total Time: 15 minutes, Serving: 4
Ingredients: 2 cups mixed berries (such as strawberries, blueberries, and raspberries)n 2 tablespoons maple syrup or agave nectar, 2 tablespoons chia seeds, 1 teaspoon lemon juice
Directions:
1. In a saucepan, combine mixed berries and maple syrup or agave nectar.
2. Cook over medium heat, stirring occasionally, until the berries begin to break down and release their juices, about 5-7 minutes.
3. Use fork or potato masher to mash the berries to your desired consistency.
4. Stir in chia seeds and lemon juice.
5. Continue to cook for another 3-5 minutes until the jam thickens.
6. Remove from heat and let cool before transferring to a jar.
7. Refrigerate the berry chia jam for at least 1 hour before serving.
Nutritional Info (per serving): Calories: 100 Protein: 2g Carbohydrates: 20g Fat: 3g Fiber: 8g

Chocolate Protein Smoothie

A rich and creamy smoothie made with banana, cocoa powder, almond milk, and protein powder, perfect for a satisfying dessert or post-workout snack.

Preparation Time: 5 minutes, Cooking Time: 0 minutes, Total Time: 5 minutes, serving: 1

Ingredients: 1 ripe banana, 1 tablespoon cocoa powder,1 scoop protein powder (chocolate flavored), 1 cup almond milk, 1/2 cup ice cubes

Directions:

1. In a blender, combine ripe banana, cocoa powder, protein powder, almond milk, and ice cubes.

2. Blend until smooth and creamy.

3. Pour the chocolate protein smoothie into a glass and serve immediately.

Nutritional Info (per serving): Calories: 250 Protein: 20g Carbohydrates: 30g Fat: 5g Fiber: 8g

Almond Butter Banana Nice Cream

Creamy and delicious "nice cream" made with frozen bananas and almond butter, perfect for a guilt-free dessert.

Preparation Time: 5 minutes, Cooking Time: 0 minutes, Total Time: 5 minutes, Serving Size: 2

Ingredients: 2 ripe bananas, sliced and frozen, 2 tablespoons almond butter, 1 tablespoon maple syrup or agave nectar (optional), Chopped almonds for topping (optional)

Directions:

1. In a blender or food processor, combine frozen banana slices, almond butter, and maple syrup or agave nectar (if using).

2. Blend the mixture until smooth and creamy, scraping down the sides as needed.

3. Serve immediately, topped with chopped almonds if desired.

Nutritional Info (per serving): Calories: 200 Protein: 4g Carbohydrates: 30g Fat: 8g Fiber: 5g

Pumpkin Pie Energy Bites

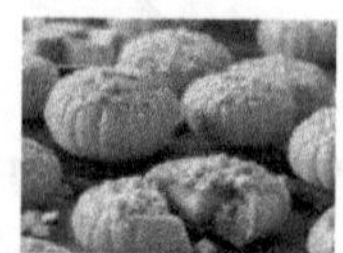

Spiced energy bites made with pumpkin puree, oats, and warming spices, perfect for a nutritious and festive treat.
Preparation Time: 10 minutes, Cooking Time: 0 minutes, Total Time: 10 minutes
Serving: 4
Ingredients: 1/2 cup pumpkin puree, 1 cup rolled oats, 1/4 cup chopped walnuts, 2 tablespoons maple syrup, 1 teaspoon pumpkin pie spice, Shredded coconut for rolling (optional)
Directions:
1. In a mixing bowl, combine pumpkin puree, rolled oats, chopped walnuts, maple syrup, and pumpkin pie spice.
2. Mix until well combined.
3. mold the mixture into small balls with your hands.
4. Optional: Roll the balls in shredded coconut for coating.
5. Refrigerate for 30 minutes before serving.
Nutritional Info (per serving): Calories: 200 Protein: 5g Carbohydrates: 25g Fat: 8g Fiber: 5g

DRESSING RECIPES

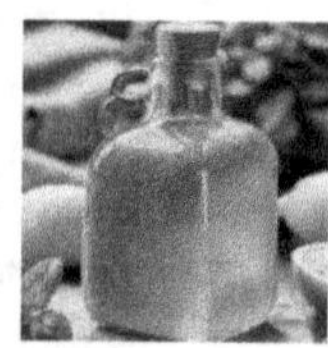

Lemon Herb Vinaigrette

Fresh and zesty, this vinaigrette bursts with the flavors of lemon and herbs.
Preparation Time: 5 minutes, Cooking Time: 0 minutes, Total Time: 5 minutes
serving: 4
Ingredients: ¼ cup lemon juice, 2 tablespoons chopped fresh herbs (such as parsley, basil, or thyme), 2 tablespoons apple cider vinegar, 1 tablespoon Dijon mustard, 1 tablespoon maple syrup, ¼ cup water
Direction:
1. Whisk all ingredients together in a bowl until well combined. Adjust sweetness or tanginess to taste.
2. Serve dressing over your favorite salads.
Nutritional Info: Calories: 15, Protein: 0g, Fat: 0g, Carbohydrates: 4g

Creamy Cashew Vinaigrette

Rich and creamy, this vinaigrette is made with protein-packed cashews for a satisfying texture.

Preparation Time: 10 minutes, Cooking Time: 0 minutes, Total Time: 10 minutes, serving: 4

Ingredients: ¼ cup raw cashews (soaked for at least 2 hours), 2 tablespoons lemon juice, 2 tablespoons apple cider vinegar, 1 tablespoon maple syrup, ½ cup water

Direction:

1. Blend all ingredients until smooth and creamy.
2. Adjust thickness with water if necessary.
3. Drizzle over salads or use as a dip for veggies.

Nutritional Info: Calories: 70, Protein: 2g, Fat: 5g, Carbohydrates: 5g

Tahini Garlic Vinaigrette

Bold and flavorful, this vinaigrette combines creamy tahini with pungent garlic.

Preparation Time: 5 minutes, Cooking Time: 0 minutes, Total Time: 5 minutes, serving: 4

Ingredients: 2 tablespoons tahini, 2 tablespoons lemon juice, 2 tablespoons apple cider vinegar, 1 clove garlic (minced), ½ cup water

Direction:

1. Whisk all ingredients together until smooth.
2. Adjust garlic intensity to taste.
3. Drizzle over roasted vegetables or salads.

Nutritional Info: Calories: 50, Protein: 2g, Fat: 4g, Carbohydrates: 3g

Soy Ginger Vinaigrette

A fusion of Asian flavors, this vinaigrette features soy sauce and ginger for a savory kick.

Preparation Time: 5 minutes, Cooking Time: 0 minutes, Total Time: 5 minutes, serving: 4

Ingredients: 2 tablespoons soy sauce (or tamari for gluten-free), 2 tablespoons rice vinegar, 1 tablespoon maple syrup, 1 teaspoon grated ginger, ½ cup water

Direction:

1. Whisk all ingredients together in a mixing bowl until well combined.
2. Adjust sweetness or tanginess if desired.
3. Drizzle over salads or use as a marinade for tofu.

Nutritional Info: Calories: 15, Protein: 1g, Fat: 0g, Carbohydrates: 3g

Chickpea Miso Vinaigrette

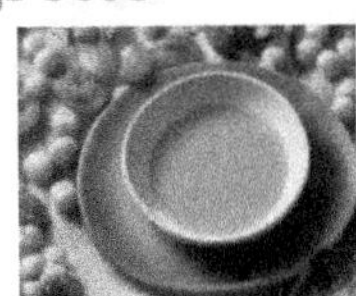

A unique twist on classic vinaigrette, this recipe incorporates the savory flavor of chickpea miso.

Preparation Time: 5 minutes, Cooking Time: 0 minutes, Total Time: 5 minutes, serving: 4

Ingredients: 2 tablespoons chickpea miso paste, 2 tablespoons rice vinegar, 1 tablespoon lemon juice, ½ cup water

Direction:
1. Whisk all ingredients together until smooth.
2. Adjust consistency with water if needed.
3. Drizzle dressing over salads or grain bowls.
Nutritional Info: Calories: 20, Protein: 2g, Fat: 0g, Carbohydrates: 3g

Hemp Seed Dill Vinaigrette

Nutty hemp seeds combined with fresh dill create a flavorful and nutritious vinaigrette.
Preparation Time: 5 minutes, Cooking Time: 0 minutes, Total Time: 5 minutes, serving: 4
Ingredients: 2 tablespoons hemp seeds, 2 tablespoons lemon juice, 2 tablespoons apple cider vinegar, 1 tablespoon chopped fresh dill, ½ cup water
Direction:
1. Blend all ingredients until smooth.
2. Adjust thickness with water if necessary.
3. Serve over salads or grilled vegetables.
Nutritional Info: Calories: 50, Protein: 3g, Fat: 3g, Carbohydrates: 3g

Creamy Avocado Cilantro Dressing

A creamy and zesty dressing perfect for salads or as a dip.
Preparation Time: 5 minutes, Cooking Time: 0 minutes, Total Time: 5 minutes, serving: 4
Ingredients: 1 ripe avocado, 1/2 cup fresh cilantro leaves, Juice of 1 lime, 1/4 cup unsweetened almond milk, 1 clove garlic
Directions:
1. In a blender, combine ripe avocado, cilantro leaves, lime juice, almond milk, and garlic.
2. Blend until smooth and creamy.
3. Adjust consistency by adding more almond milk if desired.
Nutritional Info: Calories: 80, Protein: 2g, Fat: 7g, Carbohydrates: 5g

Silken Tofu Ranch Dressing

A creamy and dairy-free take on classic ranch dressing.
Preparation Time: 5 minutes, Cooking Time: 0 minutes, Total Time: 5 minutes, serving: 4
Ingredients: 1/2 cup silken tofu, 2 tablespoons lemon juice, 1 tablespoon apple cider vinegar, 1 teaspoon dried dill,1/2 teaspoon onion powder
In a blender, combine silken tofu, lemon juice, apple cider vinegar, dried dill, and onion powder. Blend until smooth and creamy.
Nutritional Info: Calories: 30, Protein: 2g, Fat: 1g, Carbohydrates: 2g

Balsamic Maple Vinaigrette

A sweet and tangy vinaigrette perfect for drizzling over salads.
Preparation Time: 5 minutes, Cooking Time: 0 minutes, Total Time: 5 minutes, serving: 4

Ingredients: 3 tablespoons balsamic vinegar, 2 tablespoons maple syrup, 1 tablespoon Dijon mustard, 1 clove garlic, minced

Directions:

1. In a small bowl, whisk together balsamic vinegar, maple syrup, Dijon mustard, and minced garlic until well combined.

Nutritional Info: Calories: 60, Protein: 0g, Fat: 0g, Carbohydrates: 14g

Lemon Herb Greek Yogurt Dressing

A tangy and herby dressing made with protein-packed Greek yogurt.

Preparation Time: 5 minutes, Cooking Time: 0 minutes, Total Time: 5 minutes, serving: 4

Ingredients: 1/2 cup dairy-free Greek yogurt, Juice of 1 lemon, 1 tablespoon chopped fresh parsley, 1 tablespoon chopped fresh dill, 1 teaspoon honey (or maple syrup for vegan option)

Directions:

1. In a small bowl, whisk together dairy-free Greek yogurt, lemon juice, chopped fresh parsley, chopped fresh dill, and honey until well combined.

Nutritional Info: Calories: 40, Protein: 3g, Fat: 1g, Carbohydrates: 5g

Almond Butter Balsamic Vinaigrette

Creamy almond butter pairs perfectly with tangy balsamic vinegar in this satisfying vinaigrette.

Preparation Time: 5 minutes, Cooking Time: 0 minutes, Total Time: 5 minutes, serving: 4

Ingredients: 2 tablespoons almond butter, 2 tablespoons balsamic vinegar, 1 tablespoon maple syrup, ½ cup water

Direction:

1. Whisk all ingredients together until smooth.
2. Adjust sweetness to taste.
3. Drizzle over salads or roasted vegetables.

Nutritional Info: Calories: 60, Protein: 2g, Fat: 4g, Carbohydrates: 4g

Sunflower Seed Basil Vinaigrette

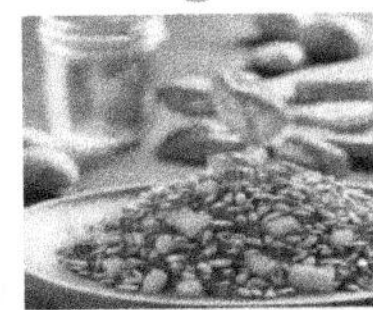

This vibrant vinaigrette combines sunflower seeds and fresh basil for a burst of flavor.

Preparation Time: 5 minutes, Cooking Time: 0 minutes, Total Time: 5 minutes, serving: 4

Ingredients: 2 tablespoons sunflower seeds, 2 tablespoons lemon juice, 2 tablespoons apple cider vinegar, 1 tablespoon chopped fresh basil, ½ cup water

Direction:

1. Blend all ingredients until well combined.
2. Adjust thickness with water if needed.

3. Drizzle over salads or grain bowls.
Nutritional Info: Calories: 50, Protein: 3g, Fat: 4g, Carbohydrates: 2g

White Bean Lemon Vinaigrette

Creamy white beans add richness to this tangy lemon vinaigrette, making it both satisfying and flavorful.

Preparation Time: 5 minutes, Cooking Time: 0 minutes, Total Time: 5 minutes, serving: 4

Ingredients: ¼ cup cooked white beans, 2 tablespoons lemon juice, 2 tablespoons apple cider vinegar, ½ cup water

Direction:

1. Blend all ingredients until smooth.
2. Adjust consistency with water if necessary.
3. Serve over salads or roasted vegetables.

Nutritional Info: Calories: 20, Protein: 1g, Fat: 0g, Carbohydrates: 4g

Pumpkin Seed Cilantro Vinaigrette

Earthy pumpkin seeds combined with fresh cilantro create a unique and flavorful vinaigrette.

Preparation Time: 5 minutes, Cooking Time: 0 minutes, Total Time: 5 minutes, serving: 4

Ingredients: 2 tablespoons pumpkin seeds, 2 tablespoons lime juice, 2 tablespoons apple cider vinegar, 1 tablespoon chopped fresh cilantro, ½ cup water

Direction:

1. Blend all ingredients until smooth.
2. Adjust seasoning to taste.
3. Drizzle dressing over salads or use as a marinade for grilled tofu.

Nutritional Info: Calories: 50, Protein: 3g, Fat: 3g, Carbohydrates: 2g

Creamy Avocado Lime Dressing

Creamy and tangy, this dressing features avocado and lime for a refreshing flavor.

Preparation Time: 5 minutes, Cooking Time: 0 minutes, Total Time: 5 minutes, serving: 4

Ingredients: 1 ripe avocado, 1 lime (juiced), 2 tablespoons apple cider vinegar, 1 tablespoon fresh cilantro (chopped), 1/4 cup water

Direction:

1. Blend all ingredients until smooth. Adjust consistency with water if needed.
2. Serve dressing over salads or roasted vegetables.

Nutritional Info: Calories: 60, Protein: 2g, Fat: 5g, Carbohydrates: 4g

Tahini Lemon Herb Dressing

Rich and aromatic, this dressing combines tahini and fresh herbs for a burst of flavor.

Preparation Time: 5 minutes, Cooking Time: 0 minutes, Total Time: 5 minutes, serving: 4

Ingredients: 2 tablespoons tahini, 1 lemon (juiced), 1 tablespoon chopped fresh herbs (such as parsley, dill, or basil), 1 clove garlic (minced), 1/4 cup water

Direction:
1. Whisk all ingredients together in a medium bowl until well combined.
2. Adjust thickness with water if necessary.
3. Drizzle dressing over salads or use as a dip for veggies.
Nutritional Info: Calories: 70, Protein: 3g, Fat: 5g, Carbohydrates: 4g

Cashew Ranch Dressing

Creamy and savory, this dressing features cashews and herbs for a classic ranch flavor.
Preparation Time: 10 minutes, Cooking Time: 0 minutes, Total Time: 10 minutes, serving: 4
Ingredients: 1/2 cup raw cashews (soaked for at least 2 hours), 2 tablespoons lemon juice, 1 tablespoon apple cider vinegar, 1 tablespoon chopped fresh chives, 1 tablespoon chopped fresh parsley, 1/4 cup water
Direction:
1. Blend all ingredients together in a blender until smooth and creamy.
2. Adjust seasoning to taste.
3. Drizzle over salads or use as a dip for raw veggies.
Nutritional Info: Calories: 80, Protein: 3g, Fat: 6g, Carbohydrates: 4g

Sunflower Seed Basil Vinaigrette

Nutty and aromatic, this vinaigrette features sunflower seeds and basil for a flavorful twist.
Preparation Time: 5 minutes, Cooking Time: 0 minutes, Total Time: 5 minutes, serving: 4
Ingredients: 2 tablespoons sunflower seeds, 1/4 cup fresh basil leaves, 1 lemon (juiced), 2 tablespoons apple cider vinegar, 1/4 cup water
Direction:
1. Blend all ingredients until well combined.
2. Adjust thickness with water if necessary.
3. Serve dressing over salads or grilled vegetables.
Nutritional Info: Calories: 50, Protein: 2g, Fat: 4g, Carbohydrates: 3g

Hemp Seed Dill Dressing

Nutty and tangy, this dressing features hemp seeds and dill for a unique and flavorful combination.
Preparation Time: 5 minutes, Cooking Time: 0 minutes, Total Time: 5 minutes, serving: 4
Ingredients: 2 tablespoons hemp seeds, 1/4 cup fresh dill (chopped), 1 lemon (juiced), 1 tablespoon apple cider vinegar, 1/4 cup water
Direction:
1. Blend all ingredients until smooth. Adjust seasoning to taste.
2. Drizzle dressing over salads or use as a marinade for grilled tofu.
Nutritional Info: Calories: 60, Protein: 3g, Fat: 4g, Carbohydrates: 3g

Almond Butter Turmeric Dressing

Rich and vibrant, this dressing features almond butter and turmeric for a flavorful and nutritious option.
Preparation Time: 5 minutes, Cooking Time: 0 minutes, Total Time: 5 minutes, serving: 4
Ingredients: 2 tablespoons almond butter, 1/2 teaspoon ground turmeric, 1 lemon (juiced), 2 tablespoons apple cider vinegar, 1/4 cup water
Direction:
1. Whisk all ingredients together until smooth. Adjust seasoning to taste.
2. Drizzle over salads or roasted vegetables.
Nutritional Info: Calories: 70, Protein: 3g, Fat: 5g, Carbohydrates: 4g

Coconut Yogurt Cilantro Lime Dressing

Creamy and refreshing, this dairy-free dressing features coconut yogurt and lime for a tropical twist.
Preparation Time: 5 minutes, Cooking Time: 0 minutes, Total Time: 5 minutes
Serving: 4
Ingredients: 1/2 cup unsweetened coconut yogurt, 1 lime (juiced), 2 tablespoons chopped fresh cilantro, 1 clove garlic (minced), 1/4 cup water
Direction:
1. Whisk all ingredients together in a medium mixing bowl until well combined.
2. Adjust thickness with water if necessary.
3. Serve over salads or grilled vegetables.
Nutritional Info: Calories: 40, Protein: 2g, Fat: 2g, Carbohydrates: 4g

Mango Avocado Dressing

Sweet and creamy, this dressing features mango and avocado for a tropical flavor explosion.
Preparation Time: 5 minutes, Cooking Time: 0 minutes, Total Time: 5 minutes
Serving: 4
Ingredients: 1 ripe mango (peeled and pitted), 1 ripe avocado (peeled and pitted), 1 lime (juiced), 1/4 cup water
Direction:
1. Blend all the ingredients together in a blender until smooth and creamy. Adjust consistency with water if needed.
2. Serve the dressing over salads or grilled vegetables.
Nutritional Info: Calories: 90, Protein: 2g, Fat: 6g, Carbohydrates: 10g

Pumpkin Seed Cilantro Vinaigrette

Earthy and aromatic, this vinaigrette features pumpkin seeds and cilantro for a unique and flavorful option.
Preparation Time: 5 minutes, Cooking Time: 0 minutes, Total Time: 5 minutesServing: 4
Ingredients: 2 tablespoons pumpkin seeds, 1/4 cup fresh cilantro (chopped), 1 lime (juiced), 2 tablespoons apple cider vinegar, 1/4 cup water
Direction:

1. Blend all ingredients until well combined. Adjust thickness with water if necessary.
2. Serve the dressing over salads or grain bowls.
Nutritional Info: Calories: 50, Protein: 3g, Fat: 3g, Carbohydrates: 4g

Sesame Ginger Dressing

Aromatic and flavorful, this dressing features sesame and ginger for a classic Asian-inspired option.
Preparation Time: 5 minutes, Cooking Time: 0 minutes, Total Time: 5 minutes, serving: 4
Ingredients: 2 tablespoons sesame seeds, 1 tablespoon grated ginger, 1 lime (juiced), 2 tablespoons coconut aminos, 1/4 cup water
Direction:
1. Blend all ingredients until smooth. Adjust seasoning to taste.
2. Drizzle the dressing over salads or use as a marinade for tofu.
Nutritional Info: Calories: 60, Protein: 3g, Fat: 4g, Carbohydrates: 4g

SOUP and STEW RECIPES

These stew and soup recipes offer a variety of flavors and are packed with protein and nutrients, making them perfect for a satisfying and wholesome meal!

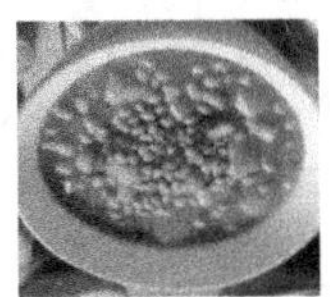

Lentil Vegetable Soup

Hearty and nutritious, this soup is loaded with lentils, vegetables, and herbs for a satisfying meal.
Preparation Time: 10 minutes, Cooking Time: 30 minutes, Total Time: 40 minutes, serving: 6
Ingredients: 1 cup dried lentils, 4 cups vegetable broth, 2 carrots (chopped), 2 celery stalks (chopped), 1 onion (chopped), 2 cloves garlic (minced), 1 teaspoon dried thyme, 1 teaspoon dried rosemary, Black pepper to taste
Direction:
1. In a large pot, combine lentils, vegetable broth, carrots, celery, onion, garlic, thyme, and rosemary.
2. Bring to a boil, then reduce heat and simmer for 25-30 minutes or until lentils are tender.
3. Season with black pepper. Serve hot and enjoy.
Nutritional Info: Calories: 180, Protein: 12g, Fat: 1g, Carbohydrates: 32g

Chickpea Spinach Soup

This flavorful soup features chickpeas and spinach in a savory broth seasoned with garlic and cumin.

Preparation Time: 10 minutes, Cooking Time: 20 minutes, Total Time: 30 minutes, Serving Size: 4

Ingredients: 1 can (15 oz) chickpeas (drained and rinsed), 4 cups vegetable broth, 2 cups fresh spinach, 1 onion (chopped), 2 cloves garlic (minced), 1 teaspoon ground cumin, 1 teaspoon paprika

Direction:

1. In a large pot, combine chickpeas, vegetable broth, spinach, onion, garlic, cumin, and paprika.
2. Bring to a simmer over low heat and let it cook for 15-20 minutes.
3. Remove from the heat and serve hot.

Nutritional Info: Calories: 160, Protein: 9g, Fat: 2g, Carbohydrates: 28g

Quinoa Vegetable Soup

Packed with protein-rich quinoa and a variety of vegetables, this soup is both nutritious and delicious.

Preparation Time: 15 minutes, Cooking Time: 25 minutes, Total Time: 40 minutes, serving: 6

Ingredients: 1/2 cup quinoa, 4 cups vegetable broth, 2 carrots (chopped), 2 celery stalks (chopped), 1 onion (chopped), 2 cloves garlic (minced), 1 zucchini (chopped), 1 teaspoon dried thyme, 1 teaspoon dried oregano

Direction:

1. In a large pot, combine quinoa, vegetable broth, carrots, celery, onion, garlic, zucchini, thyme, and oregano.
2. Bring to a boil, then reduce heat and simmer for 20-25 minutes or until quinoa is cooked and vegetables are tender.
3. Serve soup hot and enjoy!

Nutritional Info: Calories: 180, Protein: 6g, Fat: 2g, Carbohydrates: 34g

Black Bean Soup

Rich and satisfying, this soup features black beans, tomatoes, and spices for a flavorful dish.

Preparation Time: 10 minutes, Cooking Time: 30 minutes, Total Time: 40 minutes, serving: 6

Ingredients: 2 cans (15 oz each) black beans (drained and rinsed), 1 can (14.5 oz) diced tomatoes, 4 cups vegetable broth, 1 onion (chopped), 2 cloves garlic (minced), 1 teaspoon ground cumin, 1 teaspoon chili powder

Direction:

1. In a large pot, combine black beans, diced tomatoes, vegetable broth, onion, garlic, cumin, and chili powder.
2. Bring to a boil, then reduce heat and simmer for 25-30 minutes and serve hot.

Nutritional Info: Calories: 200, Protein: 12g, Fat: 1g, Carbohydrates: 36g

Split Pea Soup

Comforting and filling, this soup features split peas, carrots, and onions in a flavorful broth.
Preparation Time: 10 minutes, Cooking Time: 45 minutes, Total Time: 55 minutes, serving: 6
Ingredients: 1 1/2 cups dried split peas, 4 cups vegetable broth, 2 carrots (chopped), 1 onion (chopped), 2 cloves garlic (minced), 1 teaspoon dried thyme, 1 bay leaf
Direction:
1. In a large pot, combine split peas, vegetable broth, carrots, onion, garlic, thyme, and bay leaf.
2. Bring to a boil, then reduce heat and simmer for 40-45 minutes or until split peas are tender.
3. Remove the soup from the heat and immediately serve.
Nutritional Info: Calories: 220, Protein: 14g, Fat: 1g, Carbohydrates: 40g

Mushroom Barley Soup

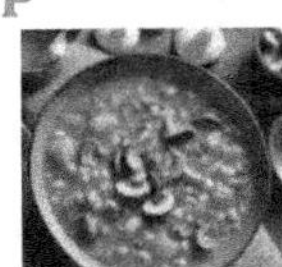

Hearty and flavorful, this soup features mushrooms, barley, and vegetables in a savory broth.
Preparation Time: 15 minutes, Cooking Time: 45 minutes, Total Time: 1 hour, serving: 6
Ingredients: 1 cup pearl barley, 4 cups vegetable broth, 2 cups sliced mushrooms, 1 onion (chopped), 2 carrots (chopped), 2 celery stalks (chopped), 2 cloves garlic (minced), 1 teaspoon dried thyme
Direction:
1. In a large pot, combine barley, vegetable broth, mushrooms, onion, carrots, celery, garlic, and thyme.
2. Bring to a boil, then reduce heat and simmer for 40-45 minutes or until barley is tender. Serve hot.
Nutritional Info: Calories: 240, Protein: 8g, Fat: 1g, Carbohydrates: 52g

Sweet Potato Lentil Soup

This hearty soup features sweet potatoes, lentils, and warming spices for a comforting meal.
Preparation Time: 15 minutes, Cooking Time: 35 minutes, Total Time: 50 minutes, serving: 6
Ingredients: 2 sweet potatoes (peeled and diced), 1 cup dried lentils, 4 cups vegetable broth, 1 onion (chopped), 2 cloves garlic (minced), 1 teaspoon ground cumin, 1/2 teaspoon ground cinnamon
Direction:
1. In a large pot, combine sweet potatoes, lentils, vegetable broth, onion, garlic, cumin, and cinnamon.
2. Bring to a boil, then reduce heat and simmer for 30-35 minutes or until sweet potatoes and lentils are tender.

3. Serve hot.
Nutritional Info: Calories: 220, Protein: 9g, Fat: 1g, Carbohydrates: 44g

Cauliflower Soup

Creamy and satisfying, this soup features cauliflower and potatoes blended with vegetable broth and herbs.

Preparation Time: 15 minutes, Cooking Time: 25 minutes, Total Time: 40 minutes, serving: 6

Ingredients: 1 head cauliflower (cut into florets), 2 potatoes (peeled and diced), 4 cups vegetable broth, 1 onion (chopped), 2 cloves garlic (minced), 1 teaspoon dried thyme, 1/2 teaspoon ground turmeric

Direction:

1. In a large pot, combine cauliflower, potatoes, vegetable broth, onion, garlic, thyme, and turmeric.

2. Bring to a boil, then reduce heat and simmer for 20-25 minutes or until vegetables are tender. Use an immersion blender to blend the soup until smooth. Serve hot.

Nutritional Info: Calories: 180, Protein: 6g, Fat: 1g, Carbohydrates: 36g

Tomato Lentil Soup

Classic and comforting, this soup features tomatoes, lentils, and vegetables in a savory broth.

Preparation Time: 10 minutes, Cooking Time: 35 minutes, Total Time: 45 minutes, serving: 6

Ingredients: 1 can (14.5 oz) diced tomatoes, 1 cup dried lentils, 4 cups vegetable broth, 1 onion (chopped), 2 carrots (chopped), 2 celery stalks (chopped), 2 cloves garlic (minced), 1 teaspoon dried basil, 1 teaspoon dried oregano

Direction:

1. In a large pot, combine diced tomatoes, lentils, vegetable broth, onion, carrots, celery, garlic, basil, and oregano.

2. Bring to a boil, then reduce heat and simmer for 30-35 minutes or until lentils are tender.

3. Serve hot.

Nutritional Info: Calories: 200, Protein: 10g, Fat: 1g, Carbohydrates: 38g

Broccoli Cauliflower Soup

Creamy and nutritious, this soup features broccoli and cauliflower blended with vegetable broth and herbs.

Preparation Time: 15 minutes, Cooking Time: 25 minutes, Total Time: 40 minutes, serving: 6

Ingredients: 1 head broccoli (cut into florets), 1 head cauliflower (cut into florets), 4 cups vegetable broth, 1 onion (chopped), 2 cloves garlic (minced), 1 teaspoon dried thyme, 1/2 teaspoon ground turmeric

Direction:

1. In a large pot, combine broccoli, cauliflower, vegetable broth, onion, garlic, thyme, and turmeric.

2. Bring to a boil, then reduce heat and simmer for 20-25 minutes or until vegetables are tender.
3. Use an immersion blender to blend until smooth. Serve hot and enjoy
Nutritional Info: Calories: 160, Protein: 8g, Fat: 1g, Carbohydrates: 32g

Hearty Lentil Stew

A comforting stew loaded with lentils, vegetables, and herbs for a nutritious meal.
Preparation Time: 15 minutes, Cooking Time: 40 minutes, Total Time: 55 minutes serving: 6
Ingredients: 1 cup dried lentils, 4 cups vegetable broth, 2 carrots (chopped), 2 celery stalks (chopped), 1 onion (chopped), 2 cloves garlic (minced), 1 teaspoon dried thyme, 1 teaspoon dried rosemary
Direction:
1. In a large pot, combine lentils, vegetable broth, carrots, celery, onion, garlic, thyme, and rosemary.
2. Bring to a boil, then reduce heat and simmer for 35-40 minutes or until lentils are tender.
3. Remove from the heat and serve immediately.
Nutritional Info: Calories: 250, Protein: 15g, Fat: 2g, Carbohydrates: 45g

Quinoa and Vegetable Stew

A protein-packed stew featuring quinoa, mixed vegetables, and savory spices for a satisfying dish.
Preparation Time: 20 minutes, Cooking Time: 30 minutes, Total Time: 50 minutes, serving: 6
Ingredients: 1/2 cup quinoa, 4 cups vegetable broth, 2 carrots (chopped), 2 celery stalks (chopped), 1 onion (chopped), 2 cloves garlic (minced), 1 zucchini (chopped), 1 teaspoon smoked paprika, 1/2 teaspoon ground cumin
Direction:
1. In a large pot, combine quinoa, vegetable broth, carrots, celery, onion, garlic, zucchini, smoked paprika, and cumin.
2. Bring to a boil, then reduce heat and simmer for 25-30 minutes or until quinoa is cooked and vegetables are tender.
3. Remove stew from heat and serve hot.
Nutritional Info: Calories: 220, Protein: 12g, Fat: 3g, Carbohydrates: 40g

Chickpea and Potato Stew

A hearty stew featuring chickpeas, potatoes, and a rich tomato base for a flavorful meal.
Preparation Time: 20 minutes, Cooking Time: 35 minutes, Total Time: 55 minutes, serving: 6
Ingredients: 2 cans (15 oz each) chickpeas (drained and rinsed), 4 cups vegetable broth, 2 potatoes (peeled and diced), 1 onion (chopped), 2 cloves garlic (minced), 1 can (14.5 oz) diced tomatoes, 1 teaspoon smoked paprika
Direction:

1. In a large pot, combine chickpeas, vegetable broth, potatoes, onion, garlic, diced tomatoes, and smoked paprika.

2. Bring to a boil, then reduce heat and simmer for 30-35 minutes or until potatoes are tender.

3. Serve hot and enjoy

Nutritional Info: Calories: 280, Protein: 14g, Fat: 2g, Carbohydrates: 50g

Red Bean and Kale Stew

A nutritious stew featuring red beans, kale, and a medley of vegetables for a comforting dish.

Preparation Time: 15 minutes, Cooking Time: 45 minutes, Total Time: 1 hour, serving: 6

Ingredients: 2 cans (15 oz each) red beans (drained and rinsed), 4 cups vegetable broth, 4 cups chopped kale, 1 onion (chopped), 2 carrots (chopped), 2 celery stalks (chopped), 2 cloves garlic (minced), 1 teaspoon dried thyme

Direction:

1. In a large pot, combine red beans, vegetable broth, kale, onion, carrots, celery, garlic, and thyme.

2. Bring to a boil, then reduce heat and simmer for 40-45 minutes or until vegetables are tender.

3. Remove soup from the heat and Serve hot.

Nutritional Info: Calories: 260, Protein: 16g, Fat: 2g, Carbohydrates: 48g

Tofu and Vegetable Stew

A protein-rich stew featuring tofu, mixed vegetables, and aromatic spices for a flavorful meal.

Preparation Time: 20 minutes, Cooking Time: 30 minutes, Total Time: 50 minutes, serving: 6

Ingredients: 1 block (14 oz) firm tofu (cubed), 4 cups vegetable broth, 2 carrots (chopped), 2 celery stalks (chopped), 1 onion (chopped), 2 cloves garlic (minced), 1 bell pepper (chopped), 1 teaspoon smoked paprika

Direction:

1. In a large pot, combine tofu, vegetable broth, carrots, celery, onion, garlic, bell pepper, and smoked paprika.

2. Bring to a boil, then reduce heat and simmer for 25-30 minutes or until vegetables are tender.

3. Serve stew hot.

Nutritional Info: Calories: 240, Protein: 18g, Fat: 4g, Carbohydrates: 35g

Mushroom and Barley Stew

A hearty stew featuring mushrooms, barley, and a savory broth for a comforting and satisfying dish.

Preparation Time: 15 minutes, Cooking Time: 40 minutes, Total Time: 55 minutes, serving: 6

Ingredients: 2 cups sliced mushrooms, 1 cup pearl barley, 4 cups vegetable broth, 1 onion (chopped), 2 carrots (chopped), 2 celery stalks (chopped), 2 cloves garlic (minced)

Direction:
1. In a large pot, combine mushrooms, barley, vegetable broth, onion, carrots, celery, and garlic.
2. Bring to a boil, then reduce heat and simmer for 35-40 minutes or until barley is tender.
3. Remove from the heat and serve hot.
Nutritional Info: Calories: 270, Protein: 14g, Fat: 2g, Carbohydrates: 50g

Spinach and Chickpea Stew

A nutritious stew featuring spinach, chickpeas, and warming spices for a flavorful and satisfying dish.
Preparation Time: 15 minutes, Cooking Time: 35 minutes, Total Time: 50 minutes, serving: 6
Ingredients: 4 cups chopped spinach, 2 cans (15 oz each) chickpeas (drained and rinsed), 1 onion (chopped), 2 cloves garlic (minced), 1 can (14.5 oz) diced tomatoes, 1 teaspoon ground cumin, 1/2 teaspoon smoked paprika
Direction:
1. In a large pot, combine spinach, chickpeas, onion, garlic, diced tomatoes, cumin, and smoked paprika. 2. Bring to a boil, then reduce heat and simmer for 30-35 minutes.
3. Remove from the heat and serve immediately.
Nutritional Info: Calories: 240, Protein: 16g, Fat: 3g, Carbohydr

Sweet Potato and Lentil Stew

A hearty stew featuring sweet potatoes, lentils, and warming spices for a comforting and nutritious meal.
Preparation Time: 20 minutes, Cooking Time: 40 minutes, Total Time: 1 hour, serving: 6
Ingredients: 2 sweet potatoes (peeled and diced), 1 cup dried green lentils, 4 cups vegetable broth, 1 onion (chopped), 2 cloves garlic (minced), 1 teaspoon ground turmeric, 1 teaspoon ground cumin
Direction:
1. In a large pot, combine sweet potatoes, lentils, vegetable broth, onion, garlic, turmeric, and cumin.
2. Bring to a boil, then reduce heat and simmer for 35-40 minutes or until sweet potatoes are tender.
3. Serve hot.
Nutritional Info: Calories: 270, Protein: 16g, Fat: 2g, Carbohydrates: 50g

Black Bean and Corn Stew

A flavorful stew featuring black beans, corn, and aromatic spices for a delicious and satisfying dish.

Preparation Time: 15 minutes, Cooking Time: 30 minutes, Total Time: 45 minutes, serving: 6

Ingredients: 2 cans (15 oz each) black beans (drained and rinsed), 1 cup corn kernels (fresh or frozen), 4 cups vegetable broth, 1 onion (chopped), 2 cloves garlic (minced), 1 teaspoon ground cumin, 1/2 teaspoon chili powder

Direction:

1. In a large pot, combine black beans, corn, vegetable broth, onion, garlic, cumin, and chili powder.
2. Bring to a boil, then reduce heat and simmer for 25-30 minutes.
3. Serve hot.

Nutritional Info: Calories: 260, Protein: 14g, Fat: 2g, Carbohydrates: 48g

Tomato and White Bean Stew

A classic stew featuring white beans, tomatoes, and Italian herbs for a flavorful and comforting meal.

Preparation Time: 15 minutes, Cooking Time: 35 minutes, Total Time: 50 minutes, serving: 6

Ingredients: 2 cans (15 oz each) white beans (drained and rinsed), 1 can (14.5 oz) diced tomatoes, 4 cups vegetable broth, 1 onion (chopped), 2 cloves garlic (minced), 1 teaspoon dried basil, 1 teaspoon dried oregano

Direction:

1. In a large pot, combine white beans, diced tomatoes, vegetable broth, onion, garlic, basil, and oregano. 2. Bring to a boil, then reduce heat and simmer over low heat for about 30-35 minutes.
3. Serve hot.

Nutritional Info: Calories: 250, Protein: 16g, Fat: 2g, Carbohydrates: 42g

SALAD RECIPES

These salads are not only delicious and satisfying but also packed with protein and nutrients, making them perfect for a nutritious meal option!

Chickpea and Spinach Salad

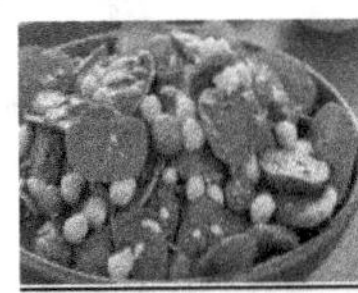

A nutrient-packed salad featuring chickpeas, fresh spinach, and a tangy lemon dressing.
Preparation Time: 10 minutes, Cooking Time: 0 minutes, Total Time: 10 minutes, serving: 2
Ingredients: 2 cups cooked chickpeas, 2 cups fresh spinach leaves, 1/4 cup sliced red onions, 1 tablespoon lemon juice, 1 tablespoon apple cider vinegar.
Direction:
1. In a large bowl, combine chickpeas, spinach, and sliced red onions.
2. Drizzle with lemon juice and apple cider vinegar.
3. Toss gently to coat and Serve immediately.
Nutritional Info: Calories: 220, Protein: 12g, Fat: 3g, Carbohydrates: 35g

Tofu and Kale Salad

A protein-rich salad featuring marinated tofu, kale, and a zesty lime dressing.
Preparation Time: 15 minutes, Cooking Time: 10 minutes, Total Time: 25 minutes, serving: 2
Ingredients: 1 block (14 oz) extra-firm tofu, 4 cups chopped kale, 1/4 cup sliced almonds, 2 tablespoons lime juice, 1 tablespoon maple syrup.
Direction:
1. Press tofu to remove excess water, then cube it.
2. Marinate tofu cubes in lime juice and maple syrup for 10 minutes.
3. In a salad bowl, combine chopped kale and sliced almonds.
4. Add marinated tofu cubes to the bowl.
5. Toss gently and serve.
Nutritional Info: Calories: 250, Protein: 18g, Fat: 10g, Carbohydrates: 25g

Black Bean and Corn Salad

A Tex-Mex inspired salad featuring black beans, sweet corn, and creamy avocado.
Preparation Time: 10 minutes, Cooking Time: 0 minutes, Total Time: 10 minutes, serving: 2
Ingredients: 1 can (15 oz) black beans (drained and rinsed), 1 cup corn kernels, 1 avocado (diced), 1/4 cup chopped cilantro, 2 tablespoons lime juice.
Direction:
1. In a large bowl, combine black beans, corn kernels, diced avocado, and chopped cilantro.
2. Drizzle with lime juice and toss gently to combine.
3. Serve chilled.
Nutritional Info: Calories: 280, Protein: 14g, Fat: 12g, Carbohydrates: 35g

Mushroom and Asparagus Salad

A flavorful salad featuring sautéed mushrooms, roasted asparagus, and mixed greens.

Preparation Time: 15 minutes, Cooking Time: 15 minutes, Total Time: 30 minutes, serving: 2

Ingredients: 2 cups mixed greens, 1 cup sliced mushrooms, 1 cup asparagus spears (trimmed), 2 tablespoons lemon juice, 1 tablespoon balsamic vinegar.

Direction:

1. Sauté sliced mushrooms until tender and roast asparagus spears in the oven until tender.
2. In a large bowl, combine mixed greens, sautéed mushrooms, and roasted asparagus.
3. Drizzle with lemon juice and balsamic vinegar.
4. Toss gently and serve.

*Nutritional Info: Calories: 180, Protein: 10g, Fat: 5g, Carbohydrates: 30g*Broccoli and

Cauliflower Salad

A crunchy salad featuring blanched broccoli and cauliflower florets, tossed in a tangy mustard dressing.

Preparation Time: 10 minutes, Cooking Time: 5 minutes, Total Time: 15 minutes, serving: 2

Ingredients: 2 cups broccoli florets (blanched), 2 cups cauliflower florets (blanched), 2 tablespoons lemon juice, 1 tablespoon Dijon mustard.

Direction:

1. In a large bowl, combine blanched broccoli and cauliflower florets.
2. In a small bowl, whisk together lemon juice and Dijon mustard.
3. Drizzle the dressing over the salad and toss to coat.
4. Serve immediately.

Nutritional Info: Calories: 160, Protein: 9g, Fat: 3g, Carbohydrates: 30g

Arugula and Beet Salad
A vibrant salad featuring peppery arugula, roasted beets, and creamy avocado.
Preparation Time: 15 minutes, Cooking Time: 45 minutes, Total Time: 60 minutes, serving: 2
Ingredients: 4 cups arugula, 2 medium beets (roasted and diced), 1 avocado (sliced), 1/4 cup sliced almonds, 2 tablespoons lemon juice.
Direction:
1. Roast beets in the oven until tender, then let them cool before dicing.
2. In a salad bowl, combine arugula, diced roasted beets, sliced avocado, and sliced almonds.
3. Drizzle with lemon juice and toss gently to combine.
4. Serve immediately and enjoy!.
Nutritional Info: Calories: 220, Protein: 8g, Fat: 15g, Carbohydrates: 30g

Bell Pepper and Cucumber Salad

A refreshing salad featuring crisp bell peppers, crunchy cucumbers, and tangy lemon dressing.
Preparation Time: 10 minutes, Cooking Time: 0 minutes, Total Time: 10 minutes, serving: 2
Ingredients: 1 red bell pepper (sliced), 1 yellow bell pepper (sliced), 1 cucumber (sliced), 2 tablespoons lemon juice, 1 tablespoon apple cider vinegar.
Direction:
1. In a large bowl, combine sliced red bell pepper, yellow bell pepper, and cucumber.
2. Drizzle with lemon juice and apple cider vinegar.
3. Toss gently to coat.
4. Serve immediately and enjoy!
Nutritional Info: Calories: 120, Protein: 4g, Fat: 2g, Carbohydrates: 25g

Tomato and Avocado Salad

A simple yet flavorful salad featuring ripe tomatoes, creamy avocado, and balsamic vinaigrette.
Preparation Time: 10 minutes, Cooking Time: 0 minutes, Total Time: 10 minutes, serving: 2
Ingredients: 2 ripe tomatoes (sliced), 1 avocado (diced), 1/4 cup chopped fresh basil, 2 tablespoons balsamic vinegar.
Direction:
1. In a salad bowl, combine sliced tomatoes, diced avocado, and chopped fresh basil.
2. Drizzle with balsamic vinegar and toss gently to coat.
3. Serve immediately.
Nutritional Info: Calories: 180, Protein: 4g, Fat: 10g, Carbohydrates: 20g

Spinach and Strawberry Salad

A delightful salad featuring baby spinach, juicy strawberries, and crunchy walnuts.
Preparation Time: 10 minutes, Cooking Time: 0 minutes, Total Time: 10 minutes, serving: 2

Ingredients: 4 cups baby spinach, 1 cup sliced strawberries, 1/4 cup chopped walnuts, 2 tablespoons balsamic vinegar.
Direction:
1. In a large mixing bowl, combine sliced strawberries, baby spinach, and chopped walnuts.
2. Drizzle with balsamic vinegar and toss gently to coat. Serve immediately.
Nutritional Info: Calories: 160, Protein: 6g, Fat: 8g, Carbohydrates: 20g

Cabbage and Carrot Salad

A crunchy salad featuring shredded cabbage, grated carrots, and a tangy lemon-ginger dressing.
Preparation Time: 15 minutes, Cooking Time: 0 minutes, Total Time: 15 minutes, serving: 2
Ingredients: 4 cups shredded cabbage, 1 cup grated carrots, 2 tablespoons lemon juice, 1 teaspoon grated ginger.
Direction:
1. In a large mixing bowl, combine grated carrots and shredded cabbage.
2. In a small bowl, whisk together lemon juice and grated ginger.
3. Drizzle the dressing over the salad and toss to coat.
4. Serve immediately.
Nutritional Info: Calories: 140, Protein: 5g, Fat: 2g, Carbohydrates: 25g

Quinoa Black Bean Salad

A protein-packed salad featuring quinoa, black beans, and colorful vegetables, tossed in a zesty lime dressing.
Preparation Time: 15 minutes, Cooking Time: 15 minutes (for quinoa), Total Time: 30 minutes, serving: 4
Ingredients: 1 cup cooked quinoa, 1 can (15 oz) black beans (drained and rinsed), 1 red bell pepper (diced), 1 cup cherry tomatoes (halved), 1/4 cup chopped cilantro, Juice of 2 limes, 1 tablespoon olive oil (optional)
Direction:
In a large bowl, combine cooked quinoa, black beans, red bell pepper, cherry tomatoes, and cilantro.
2. in a small bowl, whisk together lime juice and olive oil. Pour dressing over the salad and toss to combine.
3. Serve salad chilled.
Nutritional Info: Calories: 250, Protein: 10g, Fat: 5g, Carbohydrates: 40g

Chickpea Avocado Salad

A creamy and satisfying salad featuring chickpeas, avocado, and crunchy vegetables, dressed in a lemon tahini dressing.
Preparation Time: 15 minutes, Cooking Time: 0 minutes, Total Time: 15 minutes, serving: 4
Ingredients: 1 can (15 oz) chickpeas (drained and rinsed), 1 avocado (diced), 1 cucumber (diced), 1/2 red onion (finely chopped), Juice of 1 lemon, 2 tablespoons tahini

Direction:

1. In a large bowl, combine chickpeas, avocado, cucumber, and red onion.
2. In a small bowl, whisk together lemon juice and tahini to make the dressing.
3. Pour the dressing over the salad and toss until coated.
4. Serve salad immediately and enjoy!

Nutritional Info: Calories: 280, Protein: 12g, Fat: 15g, Carbohydrates: 30g

Tofu Edamame Salad

A protein-rich salad featuring tofu, edamame, and crunchy vegetables, drizzled with a sesame ginger dressing.

Preparation Time: 20 minutes, Cooking Time: 10 minutes (for tofu), Total Time: 30 minutes, Serving: 4

Ingredients: 1 block (14 oz) firm tofu (pressed and cubed), 1 cup shelled edamame (cooked), 1 bell pepper (thinly sliced), 1 carrot (julienned), 2 green onions (sliced), 2 tablespoons sesame seeds

Direction:

1. In a large non-stick skillet, cook tofu cubes over medium heat until golden brown, about 8-10 minutes. 2. In a large bowl, combine cooked tofu, edamame, bell pepper, carrot, and green onions.
3. Sprinkle sesame seeds on top and serve with your favorite dressing.

Nutritional Info: Calories: 320, Protein: 20g, Fat: 15g, Carbohydrates: 25g

Healthy Cucumber Chickpea Salad

A refreshing salad featuring chickpeas, cucumbers, tomatoes, olives, and feta cheese (optional), tossed in a lemon herb dressing.

Preparation Time: 15 minutes, Cooking Time: 0 minutes, Total Time: 15 minutes, Serving:4

Ingredients: 1 can (15 oz) chickpeas (drained and rinsed), 1 cucumber (diced), 1 cup cherry tomatoes (halved), 1/4 cup Kalamata olives (pitted and sliced), 2 tablespoons crumbled feta cheese (optional), Juice of 1 lemon, 2 tablespoons extra virgin olive oil (optional), 1 tablespoon chopped fresh herbs (such as parsley, dill, or mint)

Direction:

1. In a large bowl, combine chickpeas, cucumber, tomatoes, olives, and feta cheese.
2. In a small bowl, whisk together lemon juice, olive oil, and fresh herbs to make the dressing.
3. Pour the dressing over the salad and toss to coat and serve chilled.

Nutritional Info: Calories: 280, Protein: 12g, Fat: 10g, Carbohydrates: 35g

Kale Quinoa Salad

A nutritious salad featuring massaged kale, cooked quinoa, roasted sweet potatoes, and toasted almonds, tossed in a lemon vinaigrette.

Preparation Time: 20 minutes, Cooking Time: 20 minutes (for sweet potatoes), Total Time: 40 minutes, serving: 4

Ingredients: 4 cups chopped kale, 1 cup cooked quinoa, 1 sweet potato (peeled and diced), 1/4 cup sliced almonds (toasted), Juice of 1 lemon, 2 tablespoons extra virgin olive oil (optional)

Direction:

1. Preheat the oven to 400°F (200°C). Place diced sweet potatoes on a baking sheet and roast for 20 minutes or until tender.
2. In a large bowl, massage kale with lemon juice (and olive oil if using) until wilted.
3. Add cooked quinoa, roasted sweet potatoes, and toasted almonds.
4. Toss to combine and serve warm or chilled.

Nutritional Info: Calories: 300, Protein: 10g, Fat: 10g, Carbohydrates: 45g

Tuscan White Bean Salad

A hearty salad featuring white beans, sun-dried tomatoes, olives, and fresh herbs, dressed with balsamic vinaigrette.

Preparation Time: 10 minutes, Cooking Time: 0 minutes, Total Time: 10 minutes, serving: 4

Ingredients: 2 cups cooked white beans, 1/4 cup chopped sun-dried tomatoes, 1/4 cup sliced black olives, 2 tablespoons chopped fresh basil, 2 tablespoons balsamic vinegar, 1 tablespoon extra-virgin olive oil (optional)

Directions:

1. In a large bowl, combine white beans, sun-dried tomatoes, black olives, and basil.
2. Drizzle with balsamic vinegar and olive oil, if using.
3. Toss gently to combine.

Nutritional Info: Calories: 240, Protein: 10g, Fat: 5g, Carbohydrates: 35g

Asian Edamame Salad

A vibrant salad with edamame, crunchy vegetables, and a sesame ginger dressing, topped with toasted sesame seeds.

Preparation Time: 15 minutes, Cooking Time: 5 minutes, Total Time: 20 minutes, serving: 4

Ingredients: 2 cups shelled edamame, thawed, 1 cup shredded red cabbage, 1 cup shredded carrots ,1/4 cup chopped scallions, 2 tablespoons rice vinegar, 1 tablespoon sesame oil, 1 teaspoon grated ginger, 1 tablespoon toasted sesame seeds

Directions:

1. In a large bowl, combine edamame, red cabbage, carrots, and scallions.
2. In a small bowl, whisk together rice vinegar, sesame oil, and grated ginger to make the dressing.
3. Pour the dressing over the salad and toss until coated.
4. Sprinkle with toasted sesame seeds before serving.

Nutritional Info: Calories: 260, Protein: 14g, Fat: 8g, Carbohydrates: 30g

Protein-Packed Lentil Salad

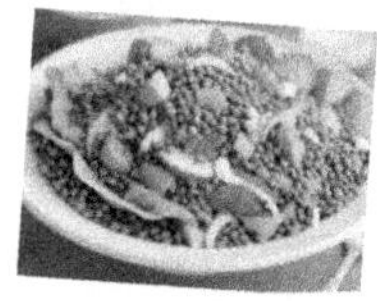

A satisfying salad with cooked lentils, crisp vegetables, and a tangy lemon tahini dressing, garnished with fresh herbs.

Preparation Time: 10 minutes, Cooking Time: 20 minutes, Total Time: 30 minutes, serving: 4

Ingredients: 1 cup cooked lentils, 1 cup diced cucumber, 1 cup diced bell pepper (any color), 1/4 cup chopped fresh parsley, 2 tablespoons tahini, Juice of 1 lemon, 1 tablespoon water

Directions:

1. In a large bowl, combine cooked lentils, cucumber, bell pepper, and parsley.
2. In a small bowl, whisk together tahini, lemon juice, and water to make the dressing.
3. Pour the dressing over the salad and toss to coat.
4. Serve garnished with additional parsley.

Nutritional Info: Calories: 280, Protein: 16g, Fat: 8g, Carbohydrates: 35g

Asian Tofu Salad

A flavorful salad featuring marinated tofu, shredded cabbage, carrots, bell peppers, and crunchy peanuts, dressed in a sesame soy dressing.

Preparation Time: 30 minutes, Cooking Time: 10 minutes (for tofu), Total Time: 40 minutes, serving: 4

Ingredients: 1 block (14 oz) firm tofu (pressed and sliced), 4 cups shredded cabbage, 1 carrot (shredded), 1 bell pepper (thinly sliced), 1/4 cup peanuts (chopped), 2 tablespoons soy sauce (or tamari), 1 tablespoon rice vinegar, 1 teaspoon sesame oil, 1 teaspoon maple syrup

Direction:

1. In a shallow dish, whisk together soy sauce, rice vinegar, sesame oil, and maple syrup.
2. Add tofu slices and let marinate for 15-20 minutes.
3. In a large skillet, cook marinated tofu over medium heat until golden brown, about 4-5 minutes per side.
4. In a large bowl, combine shredded cabbage, carrot, bell pepper, and peanuts.
5. Top with cooked tofu. Serve with your favorite dressing.

Nutritional Info: Calories: 320, Protein: 18g, Fat: 15g, Carbohydrates: 25g

Spinach Lentil Salad

A wholesome salad featuring cooked lentils, fresh spinach, cherry tomatoes, red onion, and pumpkin seeds, dressed in a balsamic vinaigrette.

Preparation Time: 15 minutes, Cooking Time: 25 minutes (for lentils), Total Time: 40 minutes, serving: 4

Ingredients: 1 cup cooked lentils, 4 cups fresh spinach leaves, 1 cup cherry tomatoes (halved), 1/4 cup thinly sliced red onion, 2 tablespoons pumpkin seeds, 2 tablespoons balsamic vinegar, 1 tablespoon Dijon mustard

Direction:

1. In a large bowl, combine cooked lentils, spinach, cherry tomatoes, red onion, and pumpkin seeds.

2. In a small bowl, whisk together balsamic vinegar and Dijon mustard to make the dressing.

3. Pour the dressing over the salad and toss to coat.

4. Serve Salad chilled and enjoy!

Nutritional Info: Calories: 250, Protein: 15g, Fat: 5g, Carbohydrates: 35g

Mango Chickpea Salad

A refreshing salad featuring chickpeas, mango, avocado, and red onion, tossed in a tangy lime dressing.

Preparation Time: 20 minutes, Cooking Time: 0 minutes, Total Time: 20 minutes, serving: 4

Ingredients: 1 can (15 oz) chickpeas (drained and rinsed), 1 ripe mango (peeled and diced), 1 avocado (diced), 1/4 cup thinly sliced red onion, Juice of 2 limes, 1 tablespoon chopped fresh cilantro

Direction:

1. In a large bowl, combine chickpeas, mango, avocado, and red onion.

2. Squeeze lime juice over the salad and sprinkle with chopped cilantro.

3. Toss gently to combine and then serve immediately.

Nutritional Info: Calories: 280, Protein: 10g, Fat: 15g, Carbohydrates: 35g

Beet and Lentil Salad

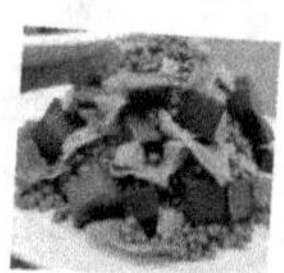

A vibrant salad featuring roasted beets, cooked lentils, arugula, and toasted walnuts, drizzled with a balsamic glaze.

Preparation Time: 20 minutes, Cooking Time: 40 minutes (for beets), Total Time: 1 hour serving: 4

Ingredients: 2 medium beets (roasted, peeled, and diced), 1 cup cooked lentils, 4 cups arugula, 1/4 cup chopped walnuts (toasted), 2 tablespoons balsamic glaze

Direction:

1. In a large bowl, combine roasted beets, cooked lentils, arugula, and toasted walnuts.

2. Drizzle with balsamic glaze and toss gently to coat.

3. Serve chilled.

Nutritional Info: Calories: 280, Protein: 12g, Fat: 10g, Carbohydrates: 40g

Greek Chickpea Salad

A Mediterranean-inspired salad featuring chickpeas, cucumber, cherry tomatoes, olives, and feta cheese (optional), dressed in a lemon herb vinaigrette.

Preparation Time: 15 minutes, Cooking Time: 0 minutes, Total Time: 15 minutes, serving: 4

Ingredients: 1 can (15 oz) chickpeas (drained and rinsed), 1 cucumber (diced), 1 cup cherry tomatoes (halved), 1/4 cup Kalamata olives (pitted and sliced), 2 tablespoons crumbled feta cheese (optional), Juice of 1 lemon, 2 tablespoons extra virgin olive oil (optional), 1 tablespoon chopped fresh herbs (such as parsley, dill, or oregano)

Direction:

1. In a large bowl, combine chickpeas, cucumber, tomatoes, olives, and feta cheese.
2. In a small bowl, whisk together lemon juice, olive oil, and fresh herbs to make the dressing.
3. Pour the dressing over the salad and toss to coat. Serve chilled.

Nutritional Info: Calories: 280, Protein: 12g, Fat: 10g, Carbohydrates: 35g

SMOOTHIE RECIPES

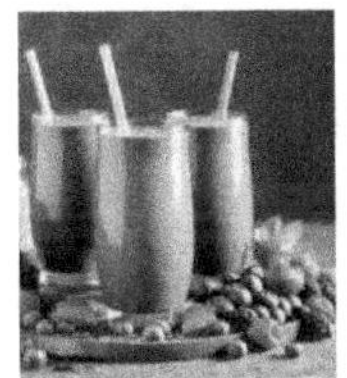

Berry Protein Power Smoothie

A delicious blend of mixed berries packed with plant-based protein to kickstart your day or refuel after a workout.

Preparation Time: 5 minutes, Cooking Time: 0 minutes, Total Time: 5 minutes, serving: 1

Ingredients: 1/2 cup mixed berries, 1/2 banana, 1/2 cup silken tofu, 1/2 cup almond milk, 1 tablespoon chia seeds.

Directions:

1. Combine all the ingredients in a blender bowl and blend until smooth and creamy.
2. Add more almond milk if needed to reach desired consistency.

Nutritional Info: Calories: 280, Protein: 12g, Fat: 10g, Carbohydrates: 35g

Green Protein Goddess Smoothie

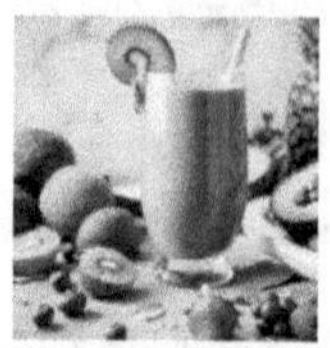

A nutrient-packed green smoothie featuring spinach and avocado, boosted with pea protein for sustained energy throughout the day.
Preparation Time: 5 minutes, Cooking Time: 0 minutes, Total Time: 5 minutes, serving: 1
Ingredients: 1 cup spinach, 1/2 avocado, 1 scoop pea protein powder, 1/2 cup almond milk, 1 tablespoon hemp seeds.
Directions:
1. Place all the ingredients in a blender bowl and blend until smooth.
2. Adjust thickness with more almond milk if desired.
Nutritional Info: Calories: 320, Protein: 15g, Fat: 12g, Carbohydrates: 25g

Chocolate Peanut Butter Protein Shake

A creamy and indulgent smoothie with the classic combination of chocolate and peanut butter, powered by plant-based protein.
Preparation Time: 5 minutes, Cooking Time: 0 minutes, Total Time: 5 minutes, Serving: 1
Ingredients: 1 tablespoon cocoa powder, 1 tablespoon natural peanut butter, 1 banana, 1/2 cup almond milk, 1 scoop chocolate plant-based protein powder.
Directions:
1. Blend all the ingredients together in blender until smooth and creamy.
2. Taste and add more almond milk if necessary to achieve desired consistency.
Nutritional Info: Calories: 300, Protein: 18g, Fat: 10g, Carbohydrates: 30g

Vanilla Almond Bliss Smoothie

A heavenly blend of almond butter and vanilla, enriched with plant-based protein for a satisfying and nourishing treat.
Preparation Time: 5 minutes, Cooking Time: 0 minutes, Total Time: 5 minutes
Serving: 1
Ingredients: 1 tablespoon almond butter, 1/2 teaspoon vanilla extract, 1 banana, 1/2 cup almond milk, 1 scoop vanilla plant-based protein powder.
Directions:
1. In a blender bowl, combine all ingredients and blend until smooth.
2. Add more almond milk if desired for consistency.
Nutritional Info: Calories: 290, Protein: 16g, Fat: 12g, Carbohydrates: 28g

Tropical Turmeric Protein Smoothie

A tropical-inspired smoothie featuring pineapple and mango, enhanced with the anti-inflammatory benefits of turmeric and plant-based protein.

Preparation Time: 5 minutes, Cooking Time: 0 minutes, Total Time: 5 minutes, serving: 1

Ingredients: 1/2 cup pineapple chunks, 1/2 cup mango chunks, 1 banana, 1/2 cup coconut water, 1 tablespoon chia seeds, 1 scoop plant-based protein powder.

Directions:

1. Add all ingredients to a blender and blend until smooth and creamy.

2. Adjust thickness with additional coconut water if needed.

Nutritional Info: Calories: 310, Protein: 14g, Fat: 8g, Carbohydrates: 40g

Berry Protein Blast Smoothie

A delicious blend of mixed berries and plant-based protein for a refreshing and nutritious smoothie.

Preparation Time: 5 minutes, Cooking Time: 0 minutes, Total Time: 5 minutes, serving: 2

Ingredients: 1 cup mixed berries (such as strawberries, blueberries, raspberries), 1 banana, frozen 1 scoop plant-based protein powder, 1 cup unsweetened almond milk

Directions:

1. Combine mixed berries, frozen banana, plant-based protein powder, and almond milk in a blender. Blend until smooth and creamy.

2. Serve smoothie immediately.

Nutritional Info: Calories: 180, Protein: 12g, Fat: 3g, Carbohydrates: 30g

Green Power Protein Smoothie

A vibrant green smoothie packed with spinach, banana, and protein for an energizing boost.

Preparation Time: 5 minutes, Cooking Time: 0 minutes, Total Time: 5 minutes,serving: 2

Ingredients: 2 cups fresh spinach, 1 banana, 1/2 avocado, 1 scoop plant-based protein powder, 1 cup unsweetened coconut water

Directions:

1. In a blender, combine fresh spinach, banana, avocado, plant-based protein powder, and coconut water. 2. Blend mixture until smooth and creamy.

3. Pour into glasses and enjoy immediately.

Nutritional Info: Calories: 220, Protein: 15g, Fat: 10g, Carbohydrates: 25g

Chocolate Peanut Butter Protein Smoothie

A decadent and satisfying smoothie featuring chocolate, peanut butter, and protein for a delightful treat.

Preparation Time: 5 minutes, Cooking Time: 0 minutes, Total Time: 5 minutes, serving: 2

Ingredients: 2 tablespoons unsweetened cocoa powder, 2 tablespoons peanut butter, 1 banana, frozen, 1 scoop plant-based chocolate protein powder, 1 cup unsweetened almond milk

Directions:

1. Add cocoa powder, peanut butter, frozen banana, plant-based chocolate protein powder, and almond milk to a blender. Blend until smooth and creamy.

2. Pour into glasses and serve immediately.

Nutritional Info: Calories: 280, Protein: 18g, Fat: 12g, Carbohydrates: 30g

Tropical Mango Protein Smoothie

A tropical delight featuring mango, pineapple, and protein for a refreshing and tropical smoothie experience.

Preparation Time: 5 minutes, Cooking Time: 0 minutes, Total Time: 5 minutes, serving: 2

Ingredients: 1 cup frozen mango chunks, 1/2 cup frozen pineapple chunks, 1 scoop plant-based vanilla protein powder, 1 cup unsweetened coconut milk

Directions:

1. Combine frozen mango chunks, frozen pineapple chunks, plant-based vanilla protein powder, and coconut milk in a blender. Blend until smooth and creamy.
2. Pour into two serving glass cup and enjoy.

Nutritional Info: Calories: 200, Protein: 14g, Fat: 3g, Carbohydrates: 35g

Creamy Almond Butter Banana Smoothie

A creamy and satisfying smoothie featuring almond butter, banana, and protein for a nourishing breakfast or snack.

Preparation Time: 5 minutes, Cooking Time: 0 minutes, Total Time: 5 minutes, serving: 2

Ingredients: 2 tablespoons almond butter, 2 bananas, frozen, 1 scoop plant-based vanilla protein powder, 1 cup unsweetened almond milk

Directions:

1. Blend almond butter, frozen bananas, plant-based vanilla protein powder, and almond milk in a blender until smooth.
2. Pour the smoothie into glasses and serve immediately.

Nutritional Info: Calories: 250, Protein: 16g, Fat: 10g, Carbohydrates: 30g

Coffee-Cacao Protein Boost Smoothie

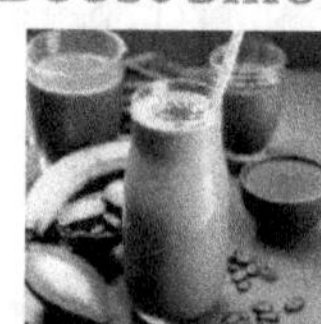

A delicious and energizing smoothie featuring the flavors of coffee and cocoa, along with plant-based protein to power you through your day.

Preparation Time: 5 minutes, Cooking Time: 0 minutes, Total Time: 5 minutes, serving: 1

Ingredients: 1/2 cup cold brew coffee, 1 banana, 1/2 cup almond milk, 1 tablespoon hemp seeds, 1 scoop plant-based protein powder.

Directions:

1. Place all the ingredients in a blender bowl and blend until smooth and creamy.
2. Add more almond milk if necessary for desired consistency.

Nutritional Info: Calories: 280, Protein: 20g, Fat: 8g, Carbohydrates: 30g

Creamy Coconut Protein Smoothie

A tropical delight with the creamy goodness of coconut, enhanced with plant-based protein for a satisfying and nourishing smoothie.

Preparation Time: 5 minutes, Cooking Time: 0 minutes, Total Time: 5 minutes, serving: 1

Ingredients: 1/2 cup coconut yogurt, 1/2 banana, 1/2 cup coconut water, 1 tablespoon shredded coconut, 1 scoop plant-based protein powder.

Directions:

1. Combine all the ingredients in a blender bowl and blend until smooth.
2. Add more coconut water if needed to reach desired consistency.

Nutritional Info: Calories: 330, Protein: 14g, Fat: 12g, Carbohydrates: 35g

Cherry Almond Chia Protein Smoothie

A refreshing smoothie with the sweetness of cherries and the nuttiness of almonds, boosted with chia seeds and plant-based protein for a nutritious drink.

Preparation Time: 5 minutes, Cooking Time: 0 minutes, Total Time: 5 minutes, serving: 1

Ingredients: 1/2 cup frozen cherries, 1 tablespoon almond butter, 1 tablespoon chia seeds, 1/2 cup almond milk, 1 scoop plant-based protein powder.

Directions:

1. Place all the ingredients in a blender bowl and blend until smooth and creamy.
2. Check the consistency of the smoothie and Adjust as needed with almond milk if desired.

Nutritional Info: Calories: 320, Protein: 16g, Fat: 10g, Carbohydrates: 30g

Minty Matcha Protein Boost Smoothie

A refreshing and invigorating smoothie featuring the vibrant flavors of matcha and mint, combined with plant-based protein for a nutritious boost.

Preparation Time: 5 minutes, Cooking Time: 0 minutes, Total Time: 5 minutes, serving: 1

Ingredients: 1 teaspoon matcha powder, a few fresh mint leaves, 1 banana, 1/2 cup almond milk, 1 tablespoon chia seeds, 1 scoop plant-based protein powder.

Directions:

1. In a blender bowl, combine all the ingredients and blend until smooth.
2. Adjust thickness with additional almond milk if needed.

Nutritional Info: Calories: 300, Protein: 15g, Fat: 10g, Carbohydrates: 35g

Pumpkin Spice Protein Smoothie

A seasonal favorite featuring the warm flavors of pumpkin spice, combined with plant-based protein for a satisfying and nourishing smoothie.

Preparation Time: 5 minutes, Cooking Time: 0 minutes, Total Time: 5 minutes, serving: 1

Ingredients: 1/2 cup pumpkin puree, 1 banana, 1/2 cup almond milk, 1 tablespoon hemp seeds, 1 scoop plant-based protein powder.

Directions:

1. Combine all the ingredients in a blender and blend until smooth.
2. Add more almond milk if necessary to achieve desired consistency.

Nutritional Info: Calories: 310, Protein: 15g, Fat: 10g, Carbohydrates: 30g

DRINK RECIPES

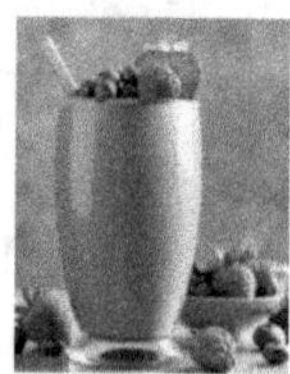

Berry Blast Protein Shake

A refreshing blend of mixed berries with plant-based protein, perfect for a quick and nutritious pick-me-up.

Preparation Time: 5 minutes, Cooking Time: 0 minutes, Total Time: 5 minutes, serving: 1

Ingredients: Mixed berries (1/2 cup), banana (1), silken tofu (1/2 cup), almond milk (1/2 cup), chia seeds (1 tablespoon).

Directions:

1. Blend all ingredients until smooth. Add more almond milk if necessary for desired consistency.

Nutritional Info: Calories: 280, Protein: 12g, Fat: 10g, Carbohydrates: 35g

Green Goddess Protein Smoothie

A nutrient-packed smoothie featuring spinach, avocado, and plant-based protein for a refreshing and energizing drink.

Preparation Time: 5 minutes, Cooking Time: 0 minutes, Total Time: 5 minutes, serving: 1

Ingredients: Spinach (1 cup), avocado (1/2), pea protein powder (1 scoop), almond milk (1/2 cup), and hemp seeds (1 tablespoon).

Directions:

1. Blend all ingredients until smooth. Adjust consistency with more almond milk if desired.

Nutritional Info: Calories: 320, Protein: 15g, Fat: 12g, Carbohydrates: 25g

Vanilla Almond Protein Shake

A creamy and delicious shake featuring the flavors of vanilla and almond, enhanced with plant-based protein for a nutritious beverage.

Preparation Time: 5 minutes, Cooking Time: 0 minutes, Total Time: 5 minutes, serving: 1

Ingredients: Almond butter (1 tablespoon), vanilla extract (1/2 teaspoon), banana (1), almond milk (1/2 cup), vanilla plant-based protein powder (1 scoop).

Directions:

1. Blend all ingredients until smooth. Add more almond milk if desired for consistency.

Nutritional Info: Calories: 290, Protein: 16g, Fat: 12g, Carbohydrates: 28g

Coffee-Cacao Protein Booster

An energizing blend of cold brew coffee, cocoa, hemp seeds, and plant-based protein for a flavorful and nutritious drink to start your day.

Preparation Time: 5 minutes, Cooking Time: 0 minutes, Total Time: 5 minutes, Serving: 1

Ingredients: Cold brew coffee (1/2 cup), banana (1), almond milk (1/2 cup), hemp seeds (1 tablespoon), plant-based protein powder (1 scoop).

Directions:

1. Combine all ingredients in a blender and blend until smooth and creamy. Adjust thickness with more almond milk if needed and serve immediately.

Nutritional Info: Calories: 280, Protein: 20g, Fat: 8g, Carbohydrates: 30g

Banana Peanut Butter Protein Smoothie

A creamy and nutty smoothie packed with protein from peanut butter and plant-based protein powder.

Preparation Time: 5 minutes, Cooking Time: 0 minutes, Total Time: 5 minutes, serving: 2

Ingredients: 2 ripe bananas, 2 tablespoons peanut butter, 1 scoop vanilla plant-based protein powder, 1 cup unsweetened almond milk

Directions:

1. Blend ripe bananas, peanut butter, vanilla plant-based protein powder, and almond milk until smooth.

2. Pour the drink into two glasses and serve immediately.

Nutritional Info: Calories: 280, Protein: 18g, Fat: 12g, Carbohydrates: 35g

Mixed Berry Protein Smoothie

A refreshing and antioxidant-rich smoothie made with mixed berries and plant-based protein powder.

Preparation Time: 5 minutes, Cooking Time: 0 minutes, Total Time: 5 minutes, serving: 2

Ingredients: *1 cup mixed berries (such as strawberries, blueberries, and raspberries), 1 scoop vanilla plant-based protein powder, 1 cup unsweetened coconut water*

Directions:

1. Blend mixed berries, vanilla plant-based protein powder, and coconut water until smooth.
2. Pour the dressing into two glasses and enjoy.
*Nutritional Info: Calories: 180, Protein: 15g, Fat: 3g, Carbohydrates: 30g*Green Protein

Power Smoothie

A nutrient-packed green smoothie loaded with spinach, banana, and protein powder for an energy boost.

Preparation Time: 5 minutes, Cooking Time: 0 minutes, Total Time: 5 minutes, serving: 2

Ingredients: 2 cups fresh spinach, 1 ripe banana, 1 scoop vanilla plant-based protein powder1 cup unsweetened almond milk

Directions:
1. Blend fresh spinach, ripe banana, vanilla plant-based protein powder, and almond milk until smooth.
2. Serve dink immediately.
Nutritional Info: Calories: 220, Protein: 16g, Fat: 10g, Carbohydrates: 25g

Chocolate Almond Protein Shake

A rich and chocolatey shake made with almond milk, cocoa powder, and protein powder for a satisfying drink.

Preparation Time: 5 minutes, Cooking Time: 0 minutes, Total Time: 5 minutes serving: 2

Ingredients: 1 cup unsweetened almond milk, 2 tablespoons unsweetened cocoa powder, 1 scoop chocolate plant-based protein powder, 1 frozen banana

Directions:
1. Blend almond milk, cocoa powder, chocolate plant-based protein powder, and frozen banana until smooth.
2. Pour the drink into two glasses and serve immediately.
Nutritional Info: Calories: 290, Protein: 20g, Fat: 14g, Carbohydrates: 30g

Coconut Pineapple Protein Smoothie

A tropical-inspired smoothie featuring pineapple, coconut milk, and protein powder for a refreshing and nutritious drink.

Preparation Time: 5 minutes, Cooking Time: 0 minutes, Total Time: 5 minutes, serving: 2

Ingredients: 1 cup frozen pineapple chunks, 1/2 cup unsweetened coconut milk, 1 scoop vanilla plant-based protein powder

Directions:
1. Blend frozen pineapple chunks, unsweetened coconut milk, and vanilla plant-based protein powder until smooth.
2. Pour the drink into two glasses and serve immediately.
Nutritional Info: Calories: 220, Protein: 15g, Fat: 8g, Carbohydrates: 30g
Cherry Almond Chia Protein Shake

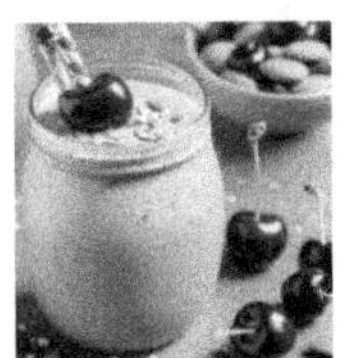

Enjoy the sweet and tangy flavors of cherries combined with the nuttiness of almonds in this protein-packed shake featuring chia seeds for an added nutritional boost.

Preparation Time: 5 minutes, Cooking Time: 0 minutes, Total Time: 5 minutes, serving: 1

Ingredients: Frozen cherries (1/2 cup), almond butter (1 tablespoon), chia seeds (1 tablespoon), almond milk (1/2 cup), plant-based protein powder (1 scoop).

Directions:

1. Blend all ingredients until creamy.

2. Adjust consistency with more almond milk if needed and enjoy.

Nutritional Info: Calories: 320, Protein: 16g, Fat: 10g, Carbohydrates: 30g

Minty Matcha Protein Booster

Refresh yourself with the invigorating flavors of matcha and mint in this protein-rich smoothie, perfect for a nutritious and energizing start to your day.

Preparation Time: 5 minutes, Cooking Time: 0 minutes, Total Time: 5 minutes, serving: 1

Ingredients: Matcha powder (1 teaspoon), fresh mint leaves (a few), banana (1), almond milk (1/2 cup), chia seeds (1 tablespoon), plant-based protein powder (1 scoop).

Directions:

1. Blend all ingredients until smooth. Add more almond milk if needed for desired consistency.

Nutritional Info: Calories: 300, Protein: 15g, Fat: 10g, Carbohydrates: 35g

SNACKS RECIPES

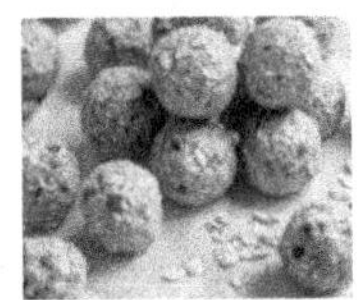

Oats Energy Bites

These energy bites are packed with nuts, seeds, and dried fruit for a satisfying snack.

Preparation Time: 15 minutes, Cooking Time: 0 minutes, Total Time: 15 minutes, serving: 12

Ingredients: 1 cup rolled oats, 1/2 cup almond butter, 1/4 cup honey or maple syrup, 1/4 cup chopped nuts (such as almonds, walnuts), 2 tablespoons chia seeds, 2 tablespoons dried cranberries or raisins

Directions:

1. In a mixing bowl, combine rolled oats, almond butter, honey or maple syrup, chopped nuts, chia seeds, and dried cranberries.
2. Mix well until everything is evenly combined.
3. Roll the mixture into small balls using your hands.
4. Place them on a baking sheet lined with parchment paper and refrigerate for at least 30 minutes before serving.
Nutritional Info: Calories: 150, Protein: 5g, Fat: 8g, Carbohydrates: 15g

Creamy Chickpea Hummus

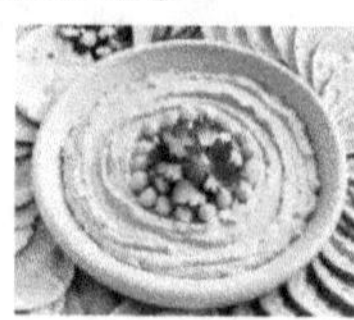

Creamy chickpea hummus served with crunchy veggie sticks for a healthy and satisfying snack.
Preparation Time: 10 minutes, Cooking Time: 0 minutes, Total Time: 10 minutes, serving: 4
Ingredients: 1 can (15 oz) chickpeas, drained and rinsed, 2 tablespoons tahini, Juice of 1 lemon, 2 cloves garlic, minced, 2 tablespoons water, Assorted vegetable sticks (carrots, cucumbers, bell peppers)
Directions:
1. In a food processor, combine chickpeas, tahini, lemon juice, minced garlic, and water.
2. Blend until smooth and creamy.
2. Serve the hummus with assorted vegetable sticks for dipping.
Nutritional Info: Calories: 120, Protein: 6g, Fat: 4g, Carbohydrates: 15g

Protein-Packed Greek Yogurt Parfait

A delicious and nutritious parfait made with dairy-free Greek yogurt, fresh fruit, and crunchy granola.
Preparation Time: 5 minutes, Cooking Time: 0 minutes, Total Time: 5 minutes, serving: 2
Ingredients: 1 cup dairy-free Greek yogurt, 1 cup mixed berries (such as strawberries, blueberries), 1/4 cup gluten-free granola, Drizzle of maple syrup (optional)
Directions:
1. In two glasses or bowls, layer dairy-free Greek yogurt, mixed berries, and gluten-free granola.
2. Drizzle with maple syrup if desired.
3. Serve immediately and enjoy.
Nutritional Info: Calories: 200, Protein: 12g, Fat: 4g, Carbohydrates: 30g

Quinoa Protein Bars

Homemade protein bars made with quinoa, nuts, seeds, and dried fruit for a nutritious snack on the go.

Preparation Time: 20 minutes, Cooking Time: 20 minutes, Total Time: 40 minutes, serving: 8

Ingredients: 1 cup cooked quinoa, 1/2 cup almond butter, 1/4 cup honey or maple syrup, 1/4 cup chopped nuts (such as almonds, cashews), 2 tablespoons chia seeds 2 tablespoons dried fruit (such as cranberries, apricots)

Directions:

1. Preheat the oven to 350°F (175°C).
2. In a large mixing bowl, combine cooked quinoa, almond butter, honey or maple syrup, chopped nuts, chia seeds, and dried fruit.
3. Mix until well combined. Press the mixture into a lined baking dish and bake for 20 minutes.
4. Let cool before cutting into bars.

Nutritional Info: Calories: 180, Protein: 6g, Fat: 8g, Carbohydrates: 20g

Rice Cake Toppers

Crunchy rice cakes topped with creamy avocado, protein-rich hummus, and sliced veggies for a satisfying snack.

Preparation Time: 5 minutes, Cooking Time: 0 minutes, Total Time: 5 minutes, serving: 2

Ingredients: 2 rice cakes (gluten-free), 1/2 avocado, sliced, 1/4 cup hummus, assorted vegetable slices (cucumbers, cherry tomatoes)

Directions:

1. Spread hummus evenly on top of each rice cake.
2. Top with sliced avocado and assorted vegetable slices.
3. Serve immediately.

Nutritional Info: Calories: 160, Protein: 6g, Fat: 8g, Carbohydrates: 20g

Protein-Packed Edamame Salad

A refreshing salad featuring edamame beans, crunchy veggies, and a tangy vinaigrette for a protein-rich snack.

Preparation Time: 10 minutes, Cooking Time: 5 minutes, Total Time: 15 minutes, serving: 4

Ingredients: 2 cups shelled edamame, cooked, 1 cup diced cucumber, 1/2 cup diced bell pepper (any color), 1/4 cup chopped fresh cilantro, Juice of 1 lime, 1 tablespoon olive oil

Directions:

1. In a large bowl, combine cooked edamame, diced cucumber, diced bell pepper, and chopped fresh cilantro.
2. Drizzle with lime juice and olive oil.
3. Toss gently to combine.
4. Serve chilled.

Nutritional Info: Calories: 140, Protein: 10g, Fat: 6g, Carbohydrates: 15g

Chickpea Salad

A protein-packed salad featuring chickpeas, fresh vegetables, and a zesty dressing.

Preparation Time: 10 minutes, Cooking Time: 0 minutes, Total Time: 10 minutes, serving: 2

Ingredients: Chickpeas (1 can, drained and rinsed), cherry tomatoes (1 cup, halved), cucumber (1, diced), red onion (1/4, finely chopped), parsley (2 tablespoons, chopped), lemon juice (2 tablespoons), olive oil (1 tablespoon, optional), black pepper (to taste).

Directions:

1. In a bowl, combine chickpeas, cherry tomatoes, cucumber, red onion, and parsley.

2. Drizzle with lemon juice (and olive oil if using), and sprinkle with black pepper.

3. Toss to combine and serve immediately.

Nutritional Info: Calories: 180, Protein: 8g, Fat: 4g, Carbohydrates: 30g

Edamame Hummus with Veggie Sticks

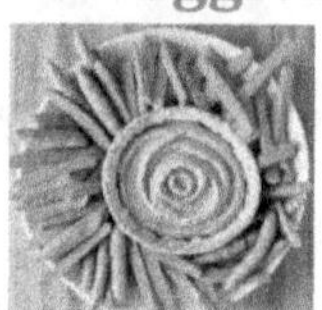

Creamy edamame hummus served with fresh vegetable sticks for a nutritious and satisfying snack.

Preparation Time: 15 minutes, Cooking Time: 5 minutes, Total Time: 20 minutes Serving: 4

Ingredients: Edamame (1 cup, shelled), tahini (2 tablespoons), lemon juice (2 tablespoons), garlic (1 clove), cumin (1/2 teaspoon), carrots (2, sliced), celery (2 stalks, sliced), bell pepper (1, sliced).

Directions:

1. Boil edamame in salt-free water for 5 minutes, then drain and cool.

2. In a food processor, combine edamame, tahini, lemon juice, garlic, and cumin.

3. Blend until smooth. Serve with vegetable sticks.

Nutritional Info: Calories: 120, Protein: 6g, Fat: 7g, Carbohydrates: 12g

Quinoa and Black Bean Salad

A hearty salad featuring quinoa, black beans, and fresh vegetables, dressed with a tangy lime vinaigrette.

Preparation Time: 15 minutes, Cooking Time: 15 minutes, Total Time: 30 minutes, serving: 4

Ingredients: Quinoa (1 cup, cooked), black beans (1 can, drained and rinsed), corn kernels (1 cup), red bell pepper (1, diced), green onions (2, chopped), cilantro (2 tablespoons, chopped), lime juice (3 tablespoons), olive oil (1 tablespoon, optional).

Directions:

1. In a large bowl, combine quinoa, black beans, corn, bell pepper, green onions, and cilantro.
2. in a small mixing bowl, whisk together lime juice and olive oil.
3. Pour the dressing over salad and toss well to coat.

Nutritional Info: Calories: 220, Protein: 10g, Fat: 4g, Carbohydrates: 35g

Protein-Packed Trail Mix

A satisfying blend of nuts, seeds, and dried fruits for a quick and nutritious snack on the go.

Preparation Time: 5 minutes, Cooking Time: 0 minutes, Total Time: 5 minutes, serving: 4

Ingredients: Almonds (1/2 cup), walnuts (1/2 cup), pumpkin seeds (1/4 cup), sunflower seeds (1/4 cup), dried cranberries (1/4 cup), dried apricots (1/4 cup, chopped).

Directions:

1. In a medium mixing bowl, combine all the ingredients and mix well.
2. Divide into individual servings and store in an airtight container.

Nutritional Info: Calories: 250, Protein: 10g, Fat: 18g, Carbohydrates: 20g

Greek Yogurt Parfait

Creamy Greek yogurt layered with fresh berries and crunchy granola for a protein-rich snack or dessert.

Preparation Time: 5 minutes, Cooking Time: 0 minutes, Total Time: 5 minutes, serving: 2

Ingredients: Greek yogurt (1 cup), mixed berries (1 cup), granola (1/2 cup, gluten-free), honey (1 tablespoon, optional).

Directions: In serving glasses or bowls, layer Greek yogurt, mixed berries, and granola. Drizzle with honey if desired.

Nutritional Info: Calories: 220, Protein: 12g, Fat: 4g, Carbohydrates: 30g

Avocado Toast

Sliced avocado on gluten-free toast, topped with tomato slices and a sprinkle of hemp seeds for a satisfying and nutritious snack.

Preparation Time: 5 minutes, Cooking Time: 5 minutes, Total Time: 10 minutes, serving: 2

Ingredients: Gluten-free bread (4 slices), avocado (1, sliced), tomato (1, sliced), hemp seeds (2 tablespoons).

Directions:
1. Toast bread slices until golden brown.
2. Top each slice with avocado slices, tomato slices, and a sprinkle of hemp seeds.
Nutritional Info: Calories: 200, Protein: 6g, Fat: 10g, Carbohydrates: 25g

Protein-Packed Energy Balls

Bite-sized energy balls made with oats, almond butter, and protein powder for a nutritious and portable snack.

Preparation Time: 15 minutes, Cooking Time: 0 minutes, Total Time: 15 minutes, serving: 12

Ingredients: Rolled oats (1 cup), almond butter (1/2 cup), honey (1/4 cup), chia seeds (2 tablespoons), plant-based protein powder (1/4 cup), shredded coconut (1/4 cup, unsweetened).

Directions:
1. In a bowl, mix together oats, almond butter, honey, chia seeds, protein powder, and shredded coconut until well combined.
2. Roll mixture into small balls.
3. Refrigerate for 30 minutes before serving.
Nutritional Info: Calories: 150, Protein: 8g, Fat: 6g, Carbohydrates: 20g

Roasted Chickpeas

Crunchy roasted chickpeas seasoned with spices for a flavorful and protein-rich snack.

Preparation Time: 10 minutes, Cooking Time: 30 minutes, Total Time: 40 minutes, serving: 4

Ingredients: Chickpeas (1 can, drained and rinsed), olive oil (1 tablespoon, optional), cumin (1 teaspoon), paprika (1 teaspoon), garlic powder (1/2 teaspoon).

Directions:
1. Preheat oven to 400°F (200°C). Pat dry the chickpeas with a paper towel.
2. In a bowl, toss chickpeas with olive oil (if using), cumin, paprika, and garlic powder.
3. Properly spread chickpeas in a single layer on a baking sheet.
4. Bake for 30 minutes, stirring halfway through, until crispy.
Nutritional Info: Calories: 180, Protein: 8g, Fat: 4g, Carbohydrates: 30g

Apple Peanut Butter Rice Cakes

Crispy rice cakes topped with creamy peanut butter and apple slices for a satisfying and protein-rich snack.

Preparation Time: 5 minutes, Cooking Time: 0 minutes, Total Time: 5 minutes, serving: 2

Ingredients: Rice cakes (4), natural peanut butter (4 tablespoons), apple (1, thinly sliced).

Directions:
1. Spread peanut butter evenly on rice cakes.
2. Top each rice cake with apple slices.
Nutritional Info: Calories: 220, Protein: 6g, Fat: 10g, Carbohydrates: 30g

APPETIZERS RECIPES

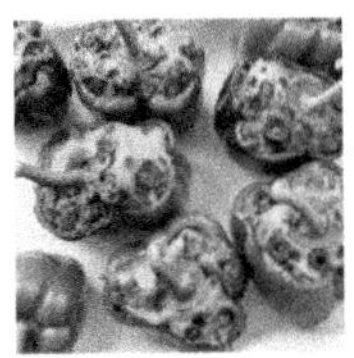

Stuffed Bell Peppers

Colorful bell peppers filled with a flavorful mixture of quinoa, black beans, and vegetables, baked to perfection.

Preparation Time: 20 minutes, Cooking Time: 25 minutes, Total Time: 45 minutes, Serving: 4

Ingredients: Bell peppers (4), quinoa (1 cup, cooked), black beans (1 can, drained and rinsed), corn kernels (1/2 cup), onion (1, diced), garlic (2 cloves, minced), cumin (1 teaspoon), chili powder (1 teaspoon), salsa (1/2 cup).

Directions:

1. Preheat oven to 375°F (190°C). In a skillet, sauté onion and garlic until soft.
2. Add cooked quinoa, black beans, corn, cumin, chili powder, and salsa.
3. Cook for 5 minutes. Stuff bell pepper halves with quinoa mixture.
4. Bake for 25 minutes until peppers are tender.

Nutritional Info: Calories: 240, Protein: 10g, Fat: 2g, Carbohydrates: 45g

Spinach and Artichoke Dip

Creamy spinach and artichoke dip made with dairy-free cream cheese and served with vegetable sticks or gluten-free crackers.

Preparation Time: 15 minutes, Cooking Time: 20 minutes, Total Time: 35 minutes, Serving: 6

Ingredients: Frozen spinach (10 oz, thawed and drained), canned artichoke hearts (1 can, drained and chopped), dairy-free cream cheese (8 oz), nutritional yeast (1/4 cup), garlic powder (1 teaspoon), lemon juice (1 tablespoon), black pepper (to taste).

Directions:

1. Preheat oven to 375°F (190°C).
2. In a mixing bowl, combine spinach, artichoke hearts, dairy-free cream cheese, nutritional yeast, garlic powder, lemon juice, and black pepper.
3. Transfer mixture to a baking dish and bake for 20 minutes until bubbly. Serve warm.

Nutritional Info: Calories: 180, Protein: 8g, Fat: 12g, Carbohydrates: 12g

Cauliflower Buffalo wings

Crispy baked cauliflower florets coated in spicy buffalo sauce, served with dairy-free ranch dip.
Preparation Time: 15 minutes, Cooking Time: 25 minutes, Total Time: 40 minutes,
Serving: 4

Ingredients: Cauliflower florets (1 head), chickpea flour (1/2 cup), almond milk (1/2 cup), garlic powder (1 teaspoon), paprika (1 teaspoon), buffalo sauce (1/2 cup), dairy-free ranch dressing (for dipping).

Directions:
1. Preheat oven to 425°F (220°C). In a bowl, whisk together chickpea flour, almond milk, garlic powder, and paprika.
2. Dip cauliflower florets into batter, then place on a baking sheet lined with parchment paper.
3. Bake for 20 minutes, flipping halfway through.
4. Remove from oven and toss in buffalo sauce.
5. Return to oven for 5 more minutes. Serve with dairy-free ranch dressing.
Nutritional Info: Calories: 180, Protein: 8g, Fat: 4g, Carbohydrates: 25g

Chickpea Hummus with Veggie Sticks

Creamy chickpea hummus paired with fresh vegetable sticks for a nutritious and protein-packed appetizer.
Preparation Time: 10 minutes, Cooking Time: 0 minutes, Total Time: 10 minutes, serving: 6

Ingredients: 1 can (15 oz) chickpeas, drained and rinsed, 2 tablespoons tahini, Juice of 1 lemon, 2 cloves garlic. 2 tablespoons water, Assorted vegetable sticks, (carrots, cucumber, bell peppers)

Directions:
1. In a food processor, blend chickpeas, tahini, lemon juice, garlic, and water until smooth.
2. Check the consistency and make an adjustment with more water if needed.
3. Serve hummus with vegetable sticks.
Nutritional Info: Calories: 120, Protein: 6g, Fat: 5g, Carbohydrates: 15g

Stuffed Mini Bell Peppers

Colorful mini bell peppers stuffed with a protein-rich filling for a delightful and healthy appetizer.
Preparation Time: 15 minutes, Cooking Time: 15 minutes, Total Time: 30 minutes, serving: 4

Ingredients: 12 mini bell peppers, 1 cup cooked quinoa, 1 can (15 oz) black beans, drained and rinsed, 1/2 cup corn kernels, 1/4 cup diced red onion, 1 teaspoon cumin

Directions:
1. Preheat oven to 375°F (190°C).
2. Cut the tops off mini bell peppers and remove seeds.
3. In a bowl, mix cooked quinoa, black beans, corn kernels, diced red onion, and cumin. Stuff each mini bell pepper with the filling.

4. Place stuffed peppers on a baking sheet and bake for 15 minutes, or until peppers are tender.
Nutritional Info: Calories: 180, Protein: 8g, Fat: 2g, Carbohydrates: 35g

Lentil Spinach Dip

A flavorful and protein-packed spin on traditional spinach dip, made with lentils for extra nutrition.

Preparation Time: 10 minutes, Cooking Time: 20 minutes, Total Time: 30 minutes, serving: 8

Ingredients: 1 cup cooked green lentils, 2 cups fresh spinach leaves, 1/2 cup dairy-free Greek yogurt, Juice of 1 lemon, 2 cloves garlic

Directions:

1. In a food processor, blend cooked green lentils, fresh spinach leaves, dairy-free Greek yogurt, lemon juice, and garlic until smooth. Adjust seasoning if needed.
2. Serve dip with vegetable sticks or gluten-free crackers.

Nutritional Info: Calories: 150, Protein: 10g, Fat: 2g, Carbohydrates: 25g

Protein-rich quinoa Stuffed Mushrooms

Juicy mushrooms stuffed with protein-rich quinoa for a savory and satisfying appetizer.

Preparation Time: 15 minutes, Cooking Time: 20 minutes, Total Time: 35 minutes, serving: 4

Ingredients: 12 large button mushrooms, 1 cup cooked quinoa, 1/2 cup diced tomatoes, 1/4 cup chopped fresh parsley, 2 tablespoons nutritional yeast

Directions:

1. Preheat oven to 375°F (190°C).
2. Remove stems from the mushrooms and set aside.
3. In a bowl, mix cooked quinoa, diced tomatoes, chopped fresh parsley, and nutritional yeast.
4. Stuff each mushroom cap with the quinoa mixture.
5. Place stuffed mushrooms on a baking sheet and bake for 20 minutes, or until mushrooms are tender.

Nutritional Info: Calories: 140, Protein: 7g, Fat: 1g, Carbohydrates: 25g

Spicy Edamame Dip

A fiery dip made with protein-packed edamame for a flavorful appetizer option.

Preparation Time: 10 minutes, Cooking Time: 5 minutes, Total Time: 15 minutes, serving: 6

Ingredients: 2 cups cooked edamame (shelled), 2 cloves garlic, Juice of 1 lime, 1 tablespoon Sriracha sauce, 2 tablespoons water

Directions:

1. In a food processor, blend cooked edamame, garlic, lime juice, Sriracha sauce, and water until smooth. Adjust spiciness according to taste.
2. Serve with gluten-free crackers or sliced vegetables.

Nutritional Info: Calories: 120, Protein: 9g, Fat: 3g, Carbohydrates: 15g

Mushroom Bruschetta

Sautéed mushrooms served on top of gluten-free baguette slices, topped with balsamic glaze and fresh basil.

Preparation Time: 15 minutes, Cooking Time: 15 minutes, Total Time: 30 minutes, serving: 6

Ingredients: Gluten-free baguette (1, sliced), mushrooms (8 oz, sliced), garlic (2 cloves, minced), balsamic vinegar (2 tablespoons), fresh basil (1/4 cup, chopped).

Directions:

1. Preheat oven to 375°F (190°C). Place baguette slices on a baking sheet and toast in the oven for 5 minutes.
2. In a skillet, sauté mushrooms and garlic until golden brown.
3. Stir in balsamic vinegar and cook for 2 more minutes.
4. Top toasted baguette slices with mushroom mixture.
5. Garnish with fresh basil.

Nutritional Info: Calories: 160, Protein: 6g, Fat: 2g, Carbohydrates: 30g

Crispy Tofu Bites

Baked tofu cubes seasoned with herbs and spices, served with a tangy dipping sauce.

Preparation Time: 15 minutes, Cooking Time: 25 minutes, Total Time: 40 minutes Serving: 4

Ingredients: Firm tofu (1 block, pressed and cubed), cornstarch (1/4 cup), nutritional yeast (1/4 cup), garlic powder (1 teaspoon), smoked paprika (1 teaspoon), tamari (2 tablespoons), maple syrup (1 tablespoon), rice vinegar (1 tablespoon), green onions (for garnish).

Directions:

1. Preheat oven to 400°F (200°C). In a bowl, combine cornstarch, nutritional yeast, garlic powder, and smoked paprika.
2. Toss tofu cubes in cornstarch mixture until coated.
3. Place tofu on a baking sheet lined with parchment paper and bake for 25 minutes, flipping halfway through.
4. In a small bowl, whisk together tamari, maple syrup, and rice vinegar.
5. Serve tofu bites with dipping sauce and garnish with chopped green onions.

Nutritional Info: Calories: 200, Protein: 12g, Fat: 6g, Carbohydrates: 20g

Avocado Cucumber Rolls

Fresh cucumber slices filled with mashed avocado, cherry tomatoes, and sprouts, drizzled with lemon juice.

Preparation Time: 15 minutes, Cooking Time: 0 minutes, Total Time: 15 minutes, serving: 4

Ingredients: Cucumber (1 large), avocado (1), cherry tomatoes (1/2 cup, halved), alfalfa sprouts (1/4 cup), lemon juice (1 tablespoon).

Directions:

1. Using a vegetable peeler, slice cucumber lengthwise into thin strips.
2. Spread mashed avocado on each cucumber slice.
3. Top with cherry tomatoes and alfalfa sprouts.

4. Drizzle with lemon juice.

5. Roll up cucumber slices and secure with toothpicks if needed.

Nutritional Info: Calories: 160, Protein: 4g, Fat: 10g, Carbohydrates: 20g

Sweet Potato Rounds with Cashew Cream

Baked sweet potato rounds topped with creamy cashew sauce and fresh herbs.

Preparation Time: 15 minutes, Cooking Time: 25 minutes, Total Time: 40 minutes, Serving: 4

Ingredients: Sweet potatoes (2, sliced into rounds), raw cashews (1 cup, soaked), lemon juice (2 tablespoons), nutritional yeast (2 tablespoons), garlic powder (1/2 teaspoon), water (1/4 cup), fresh parsley (for garnish).

Directions:

1. Preheat oven to 400°F (200°C). Place sweet potato rounds on a baking sheet lined with parchment paper and bake for 25 minutes, flipping halfway through.

2. In a blender, combine soaked cashews, lemon juice, nutritional yeast, garlic powder, and water.

3. Blend until smooth and creamy.

4. Top sweet potato rounds with cashew cream and garnish with fresh parsley.

Nutritional Info: Calories: 180, Protein: 6g, Fat: 8g, Carbohydrates: 25g

Quinoa Stuffed Mushrooms

Portobello mushroom caps filled with a savory mixture of quinoa, vegetables, and herbs, baked until golden brown.

Preparation Time: 20 minutes, Cooking Time: 25 minutes, Total Time: 45 minutes, serving: 4

Ingredients: Portobello mushrooms (4 large), quinoa (1 cup, cooked), onion (1, diced), bell pepper (1, diced), garlic (2 cloves, minced), Italian seasoning (1 teaspoon), nutritional yeast (2 tablespoons), fresh parsley (2 tablespoons, chopped).

Directions:

1. Preheat oven to 375°F (190°C). Remove stems from mushrooms and gently scrape out gills.

2. In a skillet, sauté onion, bell pepper, and garlic until softened.

3. Stir in cooked quinoa, Italian seasoning, nutritional yeast, and parsley.

4. Spoon quinoa mixture into mushroom caps.

5. Bake for 25 minutes until mushrooms are tender.

Nutritional Info: Calories: 220, Protein: 10g, Fat: 4g, Carbohydrates: 35g

Sushi Nori Wraps

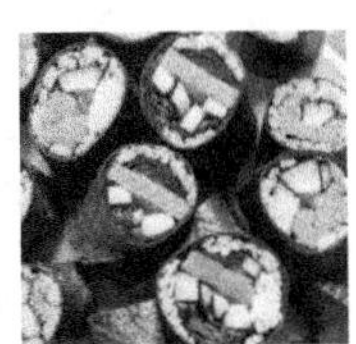

Nori seaweed sheets filled with quinoa, avocado, cucumber, and tofu, rolled into bite-sized wraps.

Preparation Time: 20 minutes, Cooking Time: 15 minutes, Total Time: 35 minutes, serving: 4

Ingredients: Nori seaweed sheets (4), quinoa (1 cup, cooked), avocado (1, sliced), cucumber (1, julienned), firm tofu (1/2 block, sliced), tamari (2 tablespoons), rice vinegar (1 tablespoon), sesame seeds (for garnish).

Directions:

1. In a skillet, sauté tofu slices in tamari and rice vinegar until golden brown.
2. Place a nori sheet on a flat surface.
3. Spread cooked quinoa on the bottom half of the nori sheet.
4. Top with avocado, cucumber, and tofu slices.
5 Roll tightly into a wrap.
6. Repeat with remaining ingredients.
7. Slice wraps into bite-sized pieces and sprinkle with sesame seeds.

Nutritional Info: Calories: 220, Protein: 12g, Fat: 8g, Carbohydrates: 30g

Caprese Skewers

Bite-sized skewers featuring cherry tomatoes, basil leaves, and dairy-free mozzarella balls, drizzled with balsamic glaze.

Preparation Time: 15 minutes, Cooking Time: 0 minutes, Total Time: 15 minutes, serving: 4

Ingredients: Cherry tomatoes (1 cup), dairy-free mozzarella balls (1 cup), fresh basil leaves (1/2 cup), balsamic glaze (2 tablespoons).

Directions:

1. Thread cherry tomatoes, mozzarella balls, and basil leaves onto skewers.
2. Arrange skewers on a serving platter and drizzle with balsamic glaze.

Nutritional Info: Calories: 180, Protein: 8g, Fat: 12g, Carbohydrates: 10g

BREAD RECIPES:

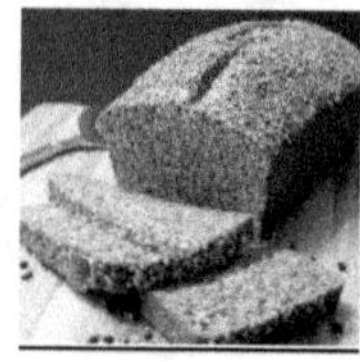

Chia Seed Bread

A hearty and nutritious bread packed with protein-rich chia seeds.

Preparation Time: 15 minutes, Cooking Time: 45 minutes, Total Time: 1 hour, Serving: 8

Ingredients: Almond flour (2 cups), chia seeds (1/4 cup), baking powder (1 tablespoon), apple cider vinegar (1 tablespoon), unsweetened almond milk (1 cup), maple syrup (2 tablespoons).

Directions:
1. Preheat oven to 350°F (175°C). In a bowl, mix almond flour, chia seeds, and baking powder.
2. Add apple cider vinegar, almond milk, and maple syrup. Stir until combined.
3. Pour batter into a greased loaf pan.
4. Bake for 45 minutes until golden brown. Allow to cool before slicing.
Nutritional Info: Calories: 180, Protein: 8g, Fat: 12g, Carbohydrates: 15g

Quinoa Flour Bread

A protein-packed bread made with quinoa flour for a nutritious and gluten-free option.
Preparation Time: 20 minutes, Cooking Time: 50 minutes, Total Time: 1 hour 10 minutes, Serving: 10
Ingredients: Quinoa flour (2 cups), baking powder (1 tablespoon), unsweetened almond milk (1 cup), apple cider vinegar (1 tablespoon), maple syrup (2 tablespoons).
Directions:
1. Preheat oven to 375°F (190°C). In a bowl, mix quinoa flour and baking powder.
2. Add almond milk, apple cider vinegar, and maple syrup. Stir until combined.
3. Pour batter into a greased loaf pan and bake for 50 minutes until a toothpick inserted into the center comes out clean.
4. Remove the bread from the oven and Let cool before slicing.
Nutritional Info: Calories: 160, Protein: 6g, Fat: 8g, Carbohydrates: 20g

Flaxseed Bread

A dense and fiber-rich bread made with flaxseeds, perfect for a high-protein snack or breakfast.
Preparation Time: 15 minutes, Cooking Time: 50 minutes, Total Time: 1 hour 5 minutes, Serving: 8
Ingredients: Ground flaxseeds (2 cups), baking powder (1 tablespoon), unsweetened almond milk (1 cup), apple cider vinegar (1 tablespoon), maple syrup (2 tablespoons).
Directions:
1. Preheat oven to 350°F (175°C). In a bowl, mix ground flaxseeds and baking powder.
2. Add almond milk, apple cider vinegar, and maple syrup. Stir until combined.
3. Pour batter into a greased loaf pan and bake for 50 minutes or until firm and golden brown.
4. Remove from the oven and Let cool before slicing.
Nutritional Info: Calories: 150, Protein: 8g, Fat: 10g, Carbohydrates: 10g

Sunflower Seed Bread

A nutty and flavorful bread made with protein-rich sunflower seeds.
Preparation Time: 20 minutes, Cooking Time: 55 minutes, Total Time: 1 hour 15 minutes , Serving: 10

Ingredients: Sunflower seed meal (2 cups), baking powder (1 tablespoon), unsweetened almond milk (1 cup), apple cider vinegar (1 tablespoon), maple syrup (2 tablespoons).
Directions:
1. Preheat oven to 375°F (190°C). In a bowl, mix sunflower seed meal and baking powder.
2. Add almond milk, apple cider vinegar, and maple syrup. Stir until combined.
3. Pour bread batter into a prepared loaf pan. Bake for 55 minutes until golden brown and firm.
4. Let cool before slicing.
Nutritional Info: Calories: 170, Protein: 10g, Fat: 12g, Carbohydrates: 10g

Hemp Seed Bread

A protein-packed bread made with hemp seeds, providing essential amino acids and omega-3 fatty acids.
Preparation Time: 20 minutes, Cooking Time: 50 minutes, Total Time: 1 hour 10 minutes, serving: 8
Ingredients: Hemp seed flour (2 cups), baking powder (1 tablespoon), unsweetened almond milk (1 cup), apple cider vinegar (1 tablespoon), maple syrup (2 tablespoons).
Directions:
1. Preheat oven to 350°F (175°C). In a bowl, mix hemp seed flour and baking powder.
2. Add almond milk, apple cider vinegar, and maple syrup. Stir until combined.
3. Pour the bread batter into a greased loaf pan.
4. Bake for 50 minutes until firm and lightly browned.
5. Remove from the oven and let cool before slicing.
Nutritional Info: Calories: 190, Protein: 12g, Fat: 14g, Carbohydrates: 10g

Almond Flour Bread

A dense and nutty bread made with almond flour, perfect for sandwiches or toast.
Preparation Time: 15 minutes, Cooking Time: 55 minutes, Total Time: 1 hour 10 minutes, Serving: 10
Ingredients: Almond flour (2 cups), baking powder (1 tablespoon), unsweetened almond milk (1 cup), apple cider vinegar (1 tablespoon), maple syrup (2 tablespoons).
Directions:
1. Preheat oven to 375°F (190°C). In a bowl, mix almond flour and baking powder.
2. Add almond milk, apple cider vinegar, and maple syrup. Stir until combined.
3. Pour batter into a greased loaf pan.
4. Bake for 55 minutes until golden brown and firm.
5. Let cool before slicing.
Nutritional Info: Calories: 180, Protein: 8g, Fat: 12g, Carbohydrates: 10g

Sesame Seed Bread

A flavorful bread made with sesame seeds, offering a crunchy texture and rich taste.

Preparation Time: 20 minutes, Cooking Time: 50 minutes, Total Time: 1 hour 10 minutes, serving: 8

Ingredients: Sesame seed meal (2 cups), baking powder (1 tablespoon), unsweetened almond milk (1 cup), apple cider vinegar (1 tablespoon), maple syrup (2 tablespoons).

Directions:

1. Preheat oven to 350°F (175°C). In a bowl, mix sesame seed meal and baking powder.
2. Add almond milk, apple cider vinegar, and maple syrup.
3. Stir until combined. Pour batter into a greased loaf pan.
4. Bake for 50 minutes until firm and lightly browned. Let cool before slicing.

Nutritional Info: Calories: 160, Protein: 10g, Fat: 10g, Carbohydrates: 10g

Pumpkin Seed Bread

A nutty and satisfying bread made with pumpkin seed meal, offering a boost of protein and essential minerals.

Preparation Time: 15 minutes, Cooking Time: 55 minutes, Total Time: 1 hour 10 minutes, serving: 10

Ingredients: Pumpkin seed meal (2 cups), baking powder (1 tablespoon), unsweetened almond milk (1 cup), apple cider vinegar (1 tablespoon), maple syrup (2 tablespoons).

Directions:

1. Preheat oven to 375°F (190°C). In a bowl, mix pumpkin seed meal and baking powder.
2. Add almond milk, apple cider vinegar, and maple syrup.
3. Stir until combined. Pour batter into a greased loaf pan.
4. Bake for 55 minutes until golden brown and firm.
5. Remove the bread from heat and let cool before slicing.

Nutritional Info: Calories: 170, Protein: 12g, Fat: 12g, Carbohydrates: 8g

Coconut Flour Bread

A light and airy bread made with coconut flour, providing a subtle coconut flavor and plenty of protein.

Preparation Time: 20 minutes, Cooking Time: 50 minutes, Total Time: 1 hour 10 minutes, serving: 8

Ingredients: Coconut flour (2 cups), baking powder (1 tablespoon), unsweetened almond milk (1 cup), apple cider vinegar (1 tablespoon), maple syrup (2 tablespoons).

Directions:

1. Preheat oven to 350°F (175°C). In a bowl, mix coconut flour and baking powder.
2. Add almond milk, apple cider vinegar, and maple syrup.
3. Stir until combined and then pour batter into a greased loaf pan.
4. Bake for 50 minutes until firm and lightly browned. Let cool before slicing.

Nutritional Info: Calories: 150, Protein: 10g, Fat: 8g, Carbohydrates: 10g

Brown Rice Flour Bread

A gluten-free and protein-rich bread made with brown rice flour, perfect for sandwiches or toast.
Preparation Time: 15 minutes, Cooking Time: 55 minutes, Total Time: 1 hour 10 minutes, serving: 10
Ingredients: Brown rice flour (2 cups), baking powder (1 tablespoon), unsweetened almond milk (1 cup), apple cider vinegar (1 tablespoon), maple syrup (2 tablespoons).
Directions:
1. Preheat oven to 375°F (190°C). In a bowl, mix brown rice flour and baking powder.
2. Add almond milk, apple cider vinegar, and maple syrup. Stir until combined.
3. Pour batter into a greased loaf pan.
4. Bake for 55 minutes until golden brown and firm.
5. Let cool before slicing.
Nutritional Info: Calories: 160, Protein: 8g, Fat: 10g, Carbohydrates: 10g

DIPS and CONDIMENT RECIPES

These high-protein plant-based dips are perfect for snacking, parties, or as appetizers. Enjoy them with your favorite dippers or as spreads for sandwiches and wraps!

Hummus

Classic chickpea-based dip with tahini and lemon juice.
Preparation Time: 10 minutes, Cooking Time: 0 minutes, Total Time: 10 minutes, serving: 6
Ingredients: 1 can (15 oz) chickpeas, 2 tablespoons tahini, 2 tablespoons lemon juice, 1 clove garlic.
Direction:
Blend all ingredients until smooth.
2. Adjust consistency with water if needed.
3. Serve with veggie sticks or pita chips.
Nutritional Info: Calories: 150, Protein: 6g, Fat: 8g, Carbohydrates: 15g

White Bean and Roasted Garlic Dip

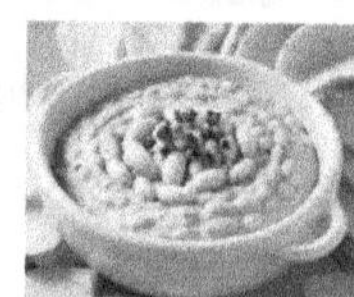

Creamy dip made with white beans and roasted garlic.
Preparation Time: 15 minutes, Cooking Time: 30 minutes, Total Time: 45 minutes, Serving: 6

Ingredients: 1 can (15 oz) white beans, 1 head garlic, 2 tablespoons lemon juice, 2 tablespoons olive oil.

Direction:

1. Roast garlic in the oven until soft.
2. Blend white beans, roasted garlic, lemon juice, and olive oil until smooth.
3. Serve with crackers or raw veggies.

Nutritional Info: Calories: 130, Protein: 5g, Fat: 7g, Carbohydrates: 15g

Edamame Dip

Vibrant dip made with edamame and fresh herbs.

Preparation Time: 10 minutes, Cooking Time: 5 minutes, Total Time: 15 minutes, serving: 6

Ingredients: 1 cup shelled edamame, 2 tablespoons lemon juice, 1 tablespoon olive oil, 2 tablespoons fresh cilantro.

Direction:

1. Cook edamame in boiling water until tender.
2. Blend with lemon juice, olive oil, and cilantro until smooth.
3. Serve dip with rice, crackers or cucumber slices.

Nutritional Info: Calories: 120, Protein: 6g, Fat: 5g, Carbohydrates: 10g

Avocado Salsa

Chunky salsa with creamy avocado and fresh tomatoes.

Preparation Time: 10 minutes, Cooking Time: 0 minutes, Total Time: 10 minutes, Serving: 6

Ingredients: 2 ripe avocados, 1 tomato (diced), 1/4 cup red onion (diced), 1 jalapeno (seeded and minced).

Direction:

1. Mash avocados in a bowl.
2. Stir in diced tomato, red onion, and minced jalapeno.
3. Serve with tortilla chips or as a topping for tacos.

Nutritional Info: Calories: 140, Protein: 3g, Fat: 10g, Carbohydrates: 10g

Avocado Hummus

Creamy hummus with a twist of avocado, perfect for dipping or spreading.

Preparation Time: 10 minutes, Cooking Time: 0 minutes, Total Time: 10 minutes, Serving: Makes about 1 1/2 cups

Ingredients: 1 ripe avocado, peeled and pitted, 1 can (15 oz) chickpeas, drained and rinsed, 2 cloves garlic, Juice of 1 lemon, 2 tablespoons tahini, 1/4 cup water

Directions:

1. In a food processor, combine avocado, garlic, tahini, chickpeas, lemon juice, and water.
2. Blend mixture until smooth and creamy. If needed, add more water to reach desired consistency.
3. Serve as a dip or spread.

Nutritional Info: Calories: 160, Protein: 6g, Fat: 8g, Carbohydrates: 18g

Vegan Pesto

Fresh and vibrant pesto made without cheese or nuts, perfect for pasta or sandwiches.
Preparation Time: 10 minutes, Cooking Time: 0 minutes, Total Time: 10 minutes, Serving: Makes about 1 cup
Ingredients: 2 cups fresh basil leaves, 1/4 cup pumpkin seeds, 2 cloves garlic, Juice of 1/2 lemon, 1/4 cup nutritional yeast, 1/4 cup water
Directions:
1. In a food processor, combine basil leaves, garlic, lemon juice, nutritional yeast, pumpkin seeds, and water.
2. Blend until smooth, stopping and scraping down the sides as needed. Adjust consistency with more water if desired.
3. Serve with pasta, salads, or sandwiches.
Nutritional Info: Calories: 120, Protein: 8g, Fat: 6g, Carbohydrates: 10g

Greek Yogurt Ranch Dressing

Creamy ranch dressing made with dairy-free Greek yogurt and flavorful herbs.
Preparation Time: 5 minutes, Cooking Time: 0 minutes, Total Time: 5 minutes, Serving: Makes about 1 cup
Ingredients: 1 cup dairy-free Greek yogurt, 2 tablespoons chopped fresh dill, 1 tablespoon chopped fresh parsley, 1 clove garlic, minced, Juice of 1/2 lemon
Directions:
1. In a small bowl, whisk together dairy-free Greek yogurt, chopped dill, chopped parsley, minced garlic, and lemon juice until well combined.
2. Taste and adjust seasoning to suit your taste.
Serve as a dressing for salads or as a dip for veggies.
Nutritional Info: Calories: 80, Protein: 6g, Fat: 2g, Carbohydrates: 8g

Spicy Mango Salsa

Refreshing salsa with a kick of spice and sweetness from fresh mango.
Preparation Time: 10 minutes, Cooking Time: 0 minutes, Total Time: 10 minutes, Serving: Makes about 2 cups
Ingredients: 2 ripe mangos, peeled and diced, 1/2 red onion, finely chopped, 1 jalapeno pepper, seeded and finely chopped, Juice of 1 lime, 2 tablespoons chopped fresh cilantro
Directions:
1. In a medium bowl, combine diced mango, chopped red onion, chopped jalapeno pepper, lime juice, and chopped cilantro. Stir well to combine.
2. Taste and make adjustment to suit your to taste.
3. Serve as a topping for grilled fish, tacos, or as a dip with tortilla chips.
Nutritional Info: Calories: 60, Protein: 2g, Fat: 0g, Carbohydrates: 15g

Sun-Dried Tomato Tapenade

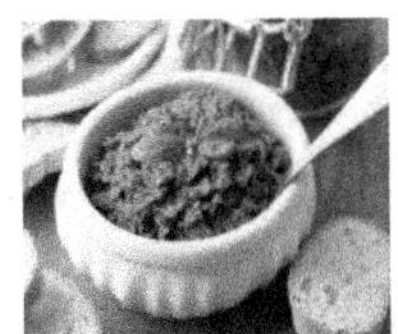

Flavorful tapenade bursting with the richness of sun-dried tomatoes.

Preparation Time: 10 minutes, Cooking Time: 0 minutes, Total Time: 10 minutes, Serving: Makes about 1 cup

Ingredients: 1 cup sun-dried tomatoes (not packed in oil), 1/4 cup toasted pine nuts, 2 cloves garlic, 2 tablespoons fresh basil leaves, Juice of 1/2 lemon

Directions:

1. In a food processor, combine sun-dried tomatoes, toasted pine nuts, garlic, basil leaves, and lemon juice.
2. Pulse until coarsely chopped and well combined. Adjust seasoning to taste.
3. Serve as a spread on crackers or crusty bread.

Nutritional Info: Calories: 100, Protein: 4g, Fat: 6g, Carbohydrates: 10g

Cilantro Lime Crema

Tangy crema with a burst of freshness from cilantro and lime, perfect for tacos or burrito bowls.

Preparation Time: 5 minutes, Cooking Time: 0 minutes, Total Time: 5 minutes, Serving: Makes about 1 cup

Ingredients: 1 cup dairy-free Greek yogurt, 1/4 cup chopped fresh cilantro, Juice of 1 lime, 1 clove garlic, minced

Directions:

1. In a small bowl, whisk together dairy-free Greek yogurt, chopped cilantro, lime juice, and minced garlic until well combined. Adjust seasoning to taste.
2. Serve as a topping for tacos, burrito bowls, or grilled vegetables.

Nutritional Info: Calories: 80, Protein: 6g, Fat: 2g, Carbohydrates: 8g

Balsamic Glaze

Sweet and tangy glaze made from balsamic vinegar, perfect for drizzling over roasted vegetables or grilled tofu.

Preparation Time: 5 minutes, Cooking Time: 10 minutes, Total Time: 15 minutes, Serving: Makes about 1/2 cup

Ingredients: 1 cup balsamic vinegar, 2 tablespoons maple syrup

Directions:

1. In a small saucepan, combine balsamic vinegar and maple syrup.
2. Bring mixture to a boil, then reduce heat to low and simmer for 8-10 minutes until the mixture is thickened and coats the back of a spoon.
3. Remove from the heat and let cool before using.
4. Drizzle over roasted vegetables, salads, or grilled tofu.

Nutritional Info: Calories: 80, Protein: 0g, Fat: 0g, Carbohydrates: 20g

Ginger-Sesame Dressing

A flavorful dressing with a hint of ginger and sesame, perfect for Asian-inspired salads or grain bowls.

Preparation Time: 5 minutes, Cooking Time: 0 minutes, Total Time: 5 minutes, Serving: Makes about 1/2 cup

Ingredients: 3 tablespoons rice vinegar, 2 tablespoons sesame oil ,1 tablespoon tamari (gluten-free soy sauce) ,1 tablespoon maple syrup, 1 teaspoon grated ginger

Directions:

1. In a small bowl, whisk together rice vinegar, sesame oil, tamari, maple syrup, and grated ginger until well combined. Adjust seasoning to taste.

2. Serve as a dressing for salads or grain bowls.

Nutritional Info: Calories: 120, Protein: 0g, Fat: 10g, Carbohydrates: 6g

Roasted Eggplant Dip

Smoky dip made with roasted eggplant and tahini.

Preparation Time: 15 minutes, Cooking Time: 30 minutes, Total Time: 45 minutes, serving: 6

Ingredients: 1 large eggplant, 2 tablespoons tahini, 2 tablespoons lemon juice, 1 clove garlic.

Direction:

1. Roast eggplant in the oven until soft.

2. Scoop out flesh and blend with tahini, lemon juice, and garlic until smooth.

3. Serve with pita bread or vegetable crudites.

Nutritional Info: Calories: 130, Protein: 4g, Fat: 8g, Carbohydrates: 15g

Black Bean Dip

Flavorful dip made with black beans, lime juice, and spices.

Preparation Time: 10 minutes, Cooking Time: 0 minutes, Total Time: 10 minutes, Serving: 6

Ingredients: 1 can (15 oz) black beans, 2 tablespoons lime juice, 1 teaspoon cumin, 1/2 teaspoon chili powder.

Direction:

1. Drain and rinse black beans.

2. Blend with lime juice, cumin, and chili powder until smooth.

3. Serve with tortilla chips or as a spread for wraps.

Nutritional Info: Calories: 140, Protein: 7g, Fat: 1g, Carbohydrates: 25g

Spinach Artichoke Dip

Creamy dip made with spinach, artichokes, and nutritional yeast.

Preparation Time: 15 minutes, Cooking Time: 15 minutes, Total Time: 30 minutes, serving: 6

Ingredients: 1 cup frozen spinach (thawed and drained), 1 can (14 oz) artichoke hearts (drained and chopped), 1/4 cup nutritional yeast, 1/4 cup dairy-free yogurt.

Direction:

1. Mix spinach, artichoke hearts, nutritional yeast, and dairy-free yogurt in a bowl.
2. Transfer to a baking dish and bake until bubbly.
3. Serve with crackers or bread.
Nutritional Info: Calories: 120, Protein: 8g, Fat: 3g, Carbohydrates: 15g

Carrot Cashew Dip

Creamy dip made with carrots, cashews, and lemon juice.
Preparation Time: 10 minutes, Cooking Time: 15 minutes, Total Time: 25 minutes. Serving: 6
Ingredients: 2 cups carrots (chopped), 1/2 cup raw cashews (soaked), 2 tablespoons lemon juice, 1 teaspoon ground cumin.
Direction:
1. Steam carrots until tender.
2. Blend carrots, soaked cashews, lemon juice, and ground cumin until smooth.
3. Serve with sliced vegetables or crackers.
Nutritional Info: Calories: 150, Protein: 5g, Fat: 8g, Carbohydrates: 15g

Cucumber Mint Yogurt Dip

Refreshing dip made with cucumber, mint, and dairy-free yogurt.
Preparation Time: 10 minutes, Cooking Time: 0 minutes, Total Time: 10 minutes, serving: 6
Ingredients: 1 cucumber (seeded and grated), 1/4 cup fresh mint (chopped), 1 cup dairy-free yogurt, 1 tablespoon lemon juice.
Direction:
1. Mix grated cucumber, chopped mint, dairy-free yogurt, and lemon juice in a bowl.
2. Chill before serving.
3. Serve with pita bread or vegetable sticks.
Nutritional Info: Calories: 130, Protein: 6g, Fat: 5g, Carbohydrates: 15g

Soy Yogurt Ranch Dip

Creamy ranch dip made with soy yogurt and herbs.
Preparation Time: 5 minutes, Cooking Time: 0 minutes, Total Time: 5 minutes, serving: 6
Ingredients: 1 cup soy yogurt, 1 tablespoon lemon juice, 1 teaspoon dried dill, 1 teaspoon dried parsley.
Direction:
1. Mix soy yogurt, lemon juice, dried dill, and dried parsley in a bowl.
2. Adjust seasoning to taste.
3. Serve with vegetable crudites or chips.
Nutritional Info: Calories: 90, Protein: 5g, Fat: 3g, Carbohydrates: 10g

BRUNCH RECIPES

These high-protein plant-based brunch recipes are delicious, nutritious, and perfect for starting your day on the right note!

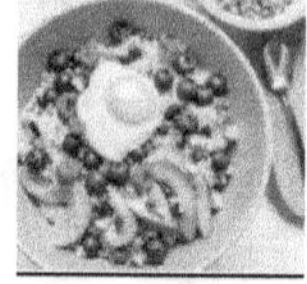

Quinoa Breakfast Bowl

A hearty bowl featuring protein-rich quinoa, avocado, and tofu scramble.
Preparation Time: 10 minutes, Cooking Time: 20 minutes, Total Time: 30 minutes, serving: 2
Ingredients: 1 cup cooked quinoa, 1 avocado (sliced), 1 cup tofu (crumbled), 1 cup mixed vegetables (such as bell peppers, onions, and spinach).
Direction:
1. Sauté mixed vegetables until tender.
2. Add crumbled tofu and cook until heated through.
3. Serve over cooked quinoa with sliced avocado on top.
Nutritional Info: Calories: 320, Protein: 15g, Fat: 15g, Carbohydrates: 30g

Healthy Chickpea Flour Pancakes

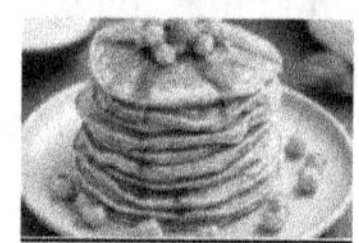

Fluffy and filling pancakes made with chickpea flour for extra protein.
Preparation Time: 10 minutes, Cooking Time: 10 minutes, Total Time: 20 minutes, serving: 2
Ingredients: 1 cup chickpea flour, 1 tablespoon flaxseed meal, 1/2 teaspoon baking powder, 1/2 cup almond milk, 1 tablespoon maple syrup.
Direction:
1. Mix all ingredients until smooth.
2. Cook on a non-stick skillet until golden brown on both sides.
3. Serve with fresh fruit or dairy-free yogurt.
Nutritional Info: Calories: 280, Protein: 12g, Fat: 8g, Carbohydrates: 40g

Tofu Scramble Wrap

Flavorful tofu scramble wrapped in a gluten-free tortilla for a satisfying brunch option.
Preparation Time: 10 minutes. Cooking Time: 10 minutes, Total Time: 20 minutes, serving: 2
Ingredients: 1 block firm tofu, 1/2 cup mixed vegetables (such as bell peppers, onions, and mushrooms), 2 gluten-free tortillas, 2 tablespoons nutritional yeast.
Direction:

1. Sauté mixed vegetables until tender.
2. Crumble tofu into the skillet and cook until heated through.
3. Sprinkle with nutritional yeast.
4. Spoon tofu scramble onto tortillas, wrap, and serve.
Nutritional Info: Calories: 240, Protein: 18g, Fat: 10g, Carbohydrates: 20g

Delicious Sweet Potato Breakfast Hash

A colorful and flavorful hash featuring sweet potatoes and black beans.
Preparation Time: 10 minutes, Cooking Time: 20 minutes, Total Time: 30 minutes, serving: 2
Ingredients: 2 medium sweet potatoes (diced), 1 can black beans (drained and rinsed), 1/2 onion (diced), 1 teaspoon smoked paprika.
Direction:
1. Roast sweet potatoes in the oven until tender.
2. Sauté onions in a skillet until translucent.
3. Add black beans and smoked paprika.
4. Stir in roasted sweet potatoes and cook until heated through.
Nutritional Info: Calories: 280, Protein: 10g, Fat: 1g, Carbohydrates: 60g

Spicy Lentil Tacos

These tacos pack a punch with spicy lentils and fresh salsa, perfect for a quick and flavorful meal.
Preparation Time: 15 minutes, Cooking Time: 25 minutes, Total Time: 40 minutes, serving: 4
Ingredients: 8 corn tortillas, 1 cup cooked lentils, 1 cup diced tomatoes, 1/4 cup diced onions, 1/4 cup chopped cilantro, 1 jalapeño (seeded and diced), 2 tablespoons lime juice, 1 teaspoon cumin, 1/2 teaspoon chili powder, 1/4 teaspoon garlic powder.
Direction:
1. In a bowl, mix cooked lentils, diced tomatoes, onions, cilantro, jalapeño, lime juice, and spices.
2. Warm tortillas and fill with lentil mixture.
3. Serve with extra salsa on top if desired. Enjoy!
Nutritional Info: Calories: 190, Protein: 8g, Fat: 4g, Carbohydrates: 30g

Veggie Tofu Frittata

A protein-packed frittata filled with colorful vegetables and tofu.
Preparation Time: 15 minutes, Cooking Time: 25 minutes, Total Time: 40 minutes, serving: 4
Ingredients: 1 block firm tofu, 1 cup mixed vegetables (such as bell peppers, spinach, and tomatoes), 1/4 cup nutritional yeast, 1 tablespoon olive oil.
Direction:
1. Sauté mixed vegetables until tender.
2. Crumble tofu into the skillet and cook until heated through.
3. Sprinkle with nutritional yeast.
4. Transfer mixture to a baking dish and bake until set. Enjoy!

Nutritional Info: Calories: 220, Protein: 15g, Fat: 10g, Carbohydrates: 15g

Chia Seed Pudding Parfait

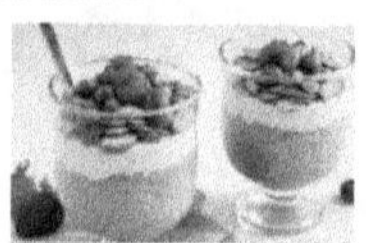

A nutritious and delicious parfait featuring chia seed pudding and fresh fruit.
Preparation Time: 5 minutes, Cooking Time: 0 minutes, Total Time: 5 minutes (+chilling time), serving: 2
Ingredients: 1/4 cup chia seeds, 1 cup almond milk, 1 tablespoon maple syrup, 1 cup mixed berries.
Direction:
1. Mix, almond milk, chia seeds and maple syrup in a bowl.
2. Let it sit in the refrigerator until thickened.
3. Layer chia seed pudding with mixed berries in glasses. Enjoy!
Nutritional Info: Calories: 200, Protein: 8g, Fat: 10g, Carbohydrates: 25g

Mushroom and Spinach Omelette

A classic omelette made with tofu instead of eggs, filled with mushrooms and spinach.
Preparation Time: 10 minutes, Cooking Time: 10 minutes, Total Time: 20 minutes, serving: 2
Ingredients: 1 block firm tofu, 1 cup sliced mushrooms, 1 cup fresh spinach, 1 tablespoon nutritional yeast.
Direction:
1. Sauté mushrooms until golden. Add spinach and cook until wilted.
2. Crumble tofu into the skillet and sprinkle with nutritional yeast.
3. Cook until heated through and serve folded.
Nutritional Info: Calories: 260, Protein: 18g, Fat: 12g, Carbohydrates: 20g

Protein-Packed Breakfast Burrito

A satisfying breakfast burrito filled with tofu scramble, black beans, and avocado.
Preparation Time: 10 minutes, Cooking Time: 10 minutes, Total Time: 20 minutes, serving: 2
Ingredients: 1 block firm tofu, 1 can black beans (drained and rinsed), 1/2 avocado (sliced), 2 gluten-free tortillas.
Direction:
1. Crumble tofu into a skillet and cook until heated through.
2. Warm black beans in a separate skillet.
3. Assemble tofu scramble, black beans, and avocado slices in tortillas.
4. Roll up and serve.
Nutritional Info: Calories: 320, Protein: 20g, Fat: 15g, Carbohydrates: 30g

Black Bean Avocado Tacos

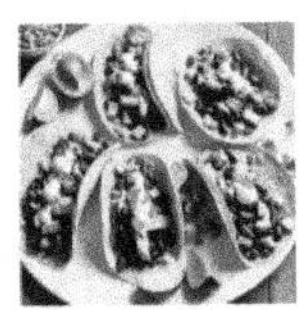

These black bean avocado tacos are a quick and easy option for a nutritious meal.
Meal Time: Anytime, Preparation Time: 15 minutes, Cooking Time: 10 minutes,
Total Time: 25 minutes, serving: 4
Ingredients: 8 corn tortillas, 1 can black beans (drained and rinsed), 1 avocado
(sliced), 1 cup diced tomatoes, 1/2 cup chopped cilantro, 1 tablespoon lime juice, 1
teaspoon cumin, 1/2 teaspoon paprika.
Direction:
1. In a skillet, warm black beans with cumin and paprika until heated through.
2. Warm corn tortillas and fill each tortilla with black beans, sliced avocado, diced
tomatoes, chopped cilantro, and a squeeze of lime juice.
Nutritional Info: Calories: 220, Protein: 9g, Fat: 8g, Carbohydrates: 30g

Protein-Packed Acai Bowl

A refreshing and nourishing acai bowl topped with granola and fruit.
**Preparation Time: 5 minutes, Cooking Time: 0 minutes, Total Time: 5
minutes Serving: 2**
Ingredients: 2 packs frozen acai puree, 1 banana, 1/2 cup mixed berries, 1/4 cup
granola.
Direction:
1. Blend acai puree with banana until smooth.
2. Pour into bowls and top with mixed berries and granola.
Nutritional Info: Calories: 280, Protein: 8g, Fat: 10g, Carbohydrates: 40g

Savory Tofu Breakfast Tacos

Flavorful breakfast tacos filled with seasoned tofu, salsa, and avocado.
Preparation Time: 10 minutes, Cooking Time: 10 minutes, Total Time: 20 minutes,
serving: 2
Ingredients: 1 block firm tofu, 1 tablespoon taco seasoning, 4 corn tortillas, 1/2
cup salsa, 1/2 avocado (sliced).
Direction:
1. Crumble tofu into a skillet and sprinkle with taco seasoning. Cook until heated
through.
2. Warm tortillas and fill with tofu scramble, salsa, and avocado slices.
Nutritional Info: Calories: 300, Protein: 18g, Fat: 12g, Carbohydrates: 30g

SAUCE RECIPES

*These sauce recipes are delicious, versatile, and perfect for enhancing the flavors of your favorite
dishes without the need for added salt, gluten, dairy, or oil. Enjoy!*

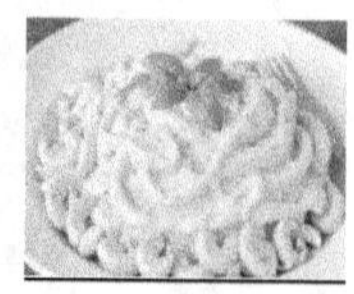

Creamy Cashew Alfredo Sauce

A velvety Alfredo sauce made with creamy cashews.
Preparation Time: 10 minutes, Cooking Time: 10 minutes, Total Time: 20 minutes, serving: 4
Ingredients: 1 cup cashews (soaked), 1 cup unsweetened almond milk, 2 tablespoons nutritional yeast, 1 clove garlic.
Direction:
1. Blend all ingredients until smooth.
2. Heat in a saucepan until warmed through.
3. Serve over pasta or steamed vegetables.
Nutritional Info: Calories: 220, Protein: 10g, Fat: 15g, Carbohydrates: 15g

Spicy Peanut Sauce

A bold and spicy sauce with the creaminess of peanut butter.
Preparation Time: 5 minutes, Cooking Time: 0 minutes, Total Time: 5 minutes, serving: 4
Ingredients: 1/4 cup peanut butter, 2 tablespoons sriracha, 2 tablespoons maple syrup, 1 tablespoon rice vinegar.
Direction:
1. Whisk all ingredients together until smooth.
2. Adjust spice level to taste.
3. Serve as a dip or sauce for stir-fries.
Nutritional Info: Calories: 180, Protein: 6g, Fat: 12g, Carbohydrates: 15g

Tahini Lemon Dressing

A tangy dressing with the nuttiness of tahini and the brightness of lemon.
Preparation Time: 5 minutes, Cooking Time: 0 minutes, Total Time: 5 minutes, serving: 4
Ingredients: 1/4 cup tahini, 1/4 cup lemon juice, 2 tablespoons water, 1 clove garlic.
Direction:
1. Whisk all ingredients together until smooth. Adjust consistency with water if needed.
2. Drizzle over salads or roasted vegetables.
Nutritional Info: Calories: 150, Protein: 4g, Fat: 10g, Carbohydrates: 10g

Roasted Red Pepper Sauce

A smoky and savory sauce made with roasted red peppers and almonds.

Preparation Time: 10 minutes, Cooking Time: 20 minutes, Total Time: 30 minutes, serving: 4

Ingredients: 2 red bell peppers, 1/4 cup almonds, 2 cloves garlic, 2 tablespoons lemon juice.

Direction:

1. Roast bell peppers in the oven until charred. Peel and remove seeds.
2. Blend with almonds, garlic, and lemon juice until smooth.
3. Heat in a saucepan until warmed through. Serve over pasta or grilled vegetables.

Nutritional Info: Calories: 180, Protein: 6g, Fat: 14g, Carbohydrates: 15g

Basil Walnut Pesto

A classic pesto with the richness of walnuts and the freshness of basil.

Preparation Time: 10 minutes, Cooking Time: 0 minutes, Total Time: 10 minutes, serving: 4

Ingredients: 2 cups fresh basil leaves, 1/2 cup walnuts, 2 cloves garlic, 1/4 cup olive oil.

Direction:

1. Blend basil, walnuts, garlic, and olive oil until smooth. Adjust seasoning to taste.
2. Serve tossed with pasta or as a spread on sandwiches.

Nutritional Info: Calories: 210, Protein: 6g, Fat: 20g, Carbohydrates: 5g

Cilantro Lime Dressing

A zesty dressing with the freshness of cilantro and lime.

Preparation Time: 5 minutes, Cooking Time: 0 minutes, Total Time: 5 minutes, serving: 4

Ingredients: 1 cup fresh cilantro leaves, 1/4 cup lime juice, 2 tablespoons olive oil, 1 clove garlic.

Direction:

1. Blend all ingredients until smooth.
2. Adjust seasoning to taste.
3. Drizzle over salads or grilled vegetables.

Nutritional Info: Calories: 170, Protein: 3g, Fat: 15g, Carbohydrates: 10g

Ginger Sesame Sauce

A flavorful sauce with the zing of ginger and the nuttiness of sesame.

Preparation Time: 5 minutes, Cooking Time: 5 minutes, Total Time: 10 minutes, serving: 4

Ingredients: 1/4 cup sesame seeds, 2 tablespoons rice vinegar, 1 tablespoon maple syrup, 1 teaspoon grated ginger.

Direction:

1. Toast sesame seeds until golden.
2. Blend with rice vinegar, maple syrup, and grated ginger until smooth.
3. Heat in a saucepan until warmed through. Serve as a dip or sauce for stir-fries.

Nutritional Info: Calories: 190, Protein: 5g, Fat: 15g, Carbohydrates: 10g

Sun-Dried Tomato Hummus

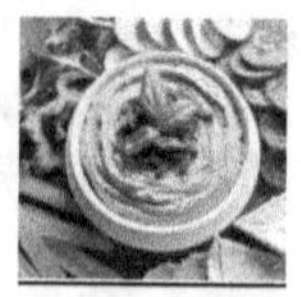

A creamy hummus with the intense flavor of sun-dried tomatoes.
Preparation Time: 10 minutes, Cooking Time: 0 minutes, Total Time: 10 minutes, serving: 4
Ingredients: 1 can (15 oz) chickpeas (drained), 1/4 cup sun-dried tomatoes (packed in oil), 2 tablespoons tahini, 2 tablespoons lemon juice.
Direction:
1. Blend all ingredients until smooth. Adjust consistency with water if needed.
2. Serve as a dip with veggies or spread on sandwiches.
Nutritional Info: Calories: 170, Protein: 7g, Fat: 8g, Carbohydrates: 20g

Mango Salsa

A fresh and fruity salsa with the sweetness of mangoes.
Preparation Time: 10 minutes, Cooking Time: 0 minutes, Total Time: 10 minutes, serving: 4
Ingredients: 2 ripe mangoes (diced), 1/4 cup red onion (diced), 1/4 cup cilantro (chopped), 1 jalapeno (seeded and minced).
Direction:
1. Mix all ingredients together in a bowl. Adjust spice level to taste.
2. Serve with tortilla chips or as a topping for grilled tofu or tempeh.
Nutritional Info: Calories: 140, Protein: 2g, Fat: 1g, Carbohydrates: 35g

Avocado Cilantro Lime Sauce

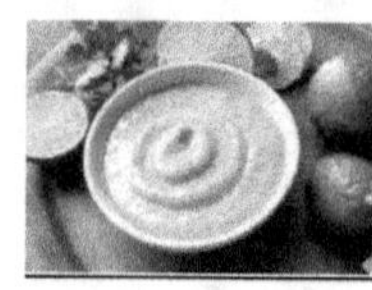

A creamy sauce with avocado, cilantro, and lime juice.
Preparation Time: 5 minutes, Cooking Time: 0 minutes, Total Time: 5 minutes, serving: 4
Ingredients: 1 ripe avocado, 1/4 cup fresh cilantro (chopped), 2 tablespoons lime juice, 2 tablespoons water.
Direction:
1. Blend avocado, cilantro, lime juice, and water until smooth.
2. Taste and adjust consistency with more water as needed.
3. Serve as a dip, sauce, or spread.
Nutritional Info: Calories: 150, Protein: 2g, Fat: 12g, Carbohydrates: 10g

CHILI RECIPES

These chili recipes are not only delicious and satisfying but also packed with protein and essential nutrients, making them perfect for a cozy meal any time of the year!

Classic Three-Bean Chili

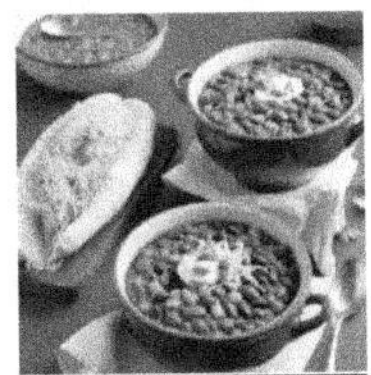

A hearty and satisfying chili packed with kidney beans, black beans, and chickpeas.
Preparation Time: 15 minutes, Cooking Time: 30 minutes, Total Time: 45 minutes, serving: 6
Ingredients: 1 can (15 oz) kidney beans, 1 can (15 oz) black beans, 1 can (15 oz) chickpeas, 1 onion (diced), 2 cloves garlic (minced), 1 can (14 oz) diced tomatoes, 2 cups vegetable broth, 2 tablespoons chili powder, 1 teaspoon cumin.
Direction:
1. In a large pot, sauté onion and garlic until soft.
2. Add beans, diced tomatoes, vegetable broth, chili powder, and cumin.
3. Simmer for 30 minutes in s low heat.
4. Serve hot and ejoy
Nutritional Info: Calories: 250, Protein: 15g, Fat: 2g, Carbohydrates: 45g

Spicy Lentil Chili

A flavorful chili made with protein-rich lentils and a blend of spices.
Preparation Time: 10 minutes, Cooking Time: 40 minutes, Total Time: 50 minutes, serving: 6
Ingredients: 1 cup green lentils, 1 onion (chopped), 2 carrots (diced), 2 celery stalks (chopped), 2 cloves garlic (minced), 1 can (14 oz) crushed tomatoes, 4 cups vegetable broth, 2 tablespoons chili powder, 1 teaspoon cumin.
Direction:
1. In a large pot, combine lentils, onion, carrots, celery, garlic, crushed tomatoes, vegetable broth, chili powder, and cumin.
2. Bring to a boil, then reduce heat and simmer for 40 minutes.
3. Serve warm.
Nutritional Info: Calories: 280, Protein: 18g, Fat: 2g, Carbohydrates: 50g

Quinoa and Black Bean Chili

A nutritious chili featuring quinoa, black beans, and a medley of vegetables.
Preparation Time: 15 minutes, Cooking Time: 30 minutes, Total Time: 45 minutes, serving: 6

Ingredients: 1 cup quinoa, 1 can (15 oz) black beans, 1 onion (chopped), 1 bell pepper (diced), 1 zucchini (chopped), 2 cloves garlic (minced), 1 can (14 oz) diced tomatoes, 2 cups vegetable broth, 2 tablespoons chili powder.

Direction:

1. In a large pot, combine quinoa, black beans, onion, bell pepper, zucchini, garlic, diced tomatoes, vegetable broth, and chili powder.
2. Simmer for 30 minutes.
3. Serve hot.

Nutritional Info: Calories: 270, Protein: 16g, Fat: 3g, Carbohydrates: 50g

Chunky Vegetable Chili

A chunky and flavorful chili loaded with assorted vegetables and beans.

Preparation Time: 20 minutes, Cooking Time: 35 minutes, Total Time: 55 minutes, serving: 6

Ingredients: 1 onion (chopped), 2 carrots (diced), 2 celery stalks (chopped), 1 bell pepper (diced), 2 cloves garlic (minced), 1 can (15 oz) kidney beans, 1 can (15 oz) pinto beans, 1 can (14 oz) diced tomatoes, 2 cups vegetable broth, 2 tablespoons chili powder.

Direction:

1. In a large pot, sauté onion, carrots, celery, bell pepper, and garlic until tender.
2. Add beans, diced tomatoes, vegetable broth, and chili powder.
3. Simmer for 35 minutes.
4. Serve warm.

Nutritional Info: Calories: 240, Protein: 14g, Fat: 2g, Carbohydrates: 45g

Sweet Potato and Lentil Chili

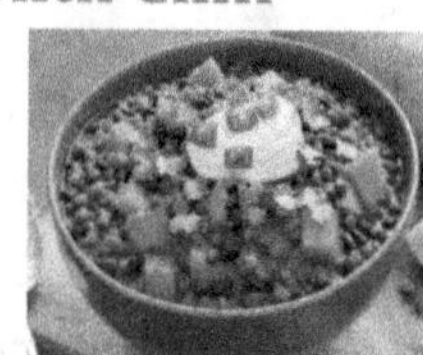

A comforting chili featuring sweet potatoes, lentils, and warming spices.

Preparation Time: 15 minutes, Cooking Time: 40 minutes, Total Time: 55 minutes, serving: 6

Ingredients: 2 sweet potatoes (peeled and diced), 1 cup green lentils, 1 onion (chopped), 2 cloves garlic (minced), 1 can (14 oz) diced tomatoes, 4 cups vegetable broth, 2 tablespoons chili powder, 1 teaspoon cumin.

Direction:

1. In a large pot, combine sweet potatoes, lentils, onion, garlic, diced tomatoes, vegetable broth, chili powder, and cumin.
2. In a low heat, simmer for 40 minutes until sweet potatoes are tender.
3. Serve hot.

Nutritional Info: Calories: 280, Protein: 14g, Fat: 1g, Carbohydrates: 55g

Mushroom and Black Bean Chili

A rich and earthy chili made with mushrooms, black beans, and aromatic spices.
Preparation Time: 20 minutes, Cooking Time: 30 minutes, Total Time: 50 minutes. Serving: 6
Ingredients: 1 onion (chopped), 2 cloves garlic (minced), 8 oz mushrooms (sliced), 1 can (15 oz) black beans, 1 can (14 oz) diced tomatoes, 2 cups vegetable broth, 2 tablespoons chili powder, 1 teaspoon cumin.
Direction:
1. In a large pot, sauté onion and garlic until fragrant.
2. Add mushrooms and cook until softened. Stir in black beans, diced tomatoes, vegetable broth, chili powder, and cumin.
3. Let it simmer for 30 minutes.
4. Remove from the heat and Serve hot.
Nutritional Info: Calories: 260, Protein: 16g, Fat: 2g, Carbohydrates: 50g

Tofu and Vegetable Chili

A protein-packed chili made with tofu, mixed vegetables, and bold spices.
Preparation Time: 20 minutes, Cooking Time: 30 minutes, Total Time: 50 minutes. Serving: 6
Ingredients: 1 block (14 oz) tofu (firm or extra firm, diced), 1 onion (chopped), 1 bell pepper (diced), 1 zucchini (chopped), 2 cloves garlic (minced), 1 can (15 oz) kidney beans, 1 can (15 oz) diced tomatoes, 2 cups vegetable broth, 2 tablespoons chili powder.
Direction:
1. In a large pot, sauté tofu, onion, bell pepper, zucchini, and garlic until vegetables are tender.
2. Add kidney beans, diced tomatoes, vegetable broth, and chili powder.
3. Simmer for 30 minutes over low heat.
4. Serve warm and enjoy!
Nutritional Info: Calories: 270, Protein: 18g, Fat: 4g, Carbohydrates: 45g

Corn and Black-Eyed Pea Chili

A comforting chili featuring sweet corn, black-eyed peas, and Tex-Mex flavors.
Preparation Time: 15 minutes, Cooking Time: 35 minutes, Total Time: 50 minutes, serving: 6
Ingredients: 2 cups frozen corn kernels, 1 can (15 oz) black-eyed peas, 1 onion (chopped), 1 bell pepper (diced), 2 cloves garlic (minced), 1 can (14 oz) diced tomatoes, 2 cups vegetable broth, 2 tablespoons chili powder, 1 teaspoon cumin.
Direction:
1. In a large pot, sauté onion, bell pepper, and garlic until softened.
2. Add corn kernels, black-eyed peas, diced tomatoes, vegetable broth, chili powder, and cumin.
3. Simmer for 35 minutes over low heat and serve hot.enjoy
Nutritional Info: Calories: 260, Protein: 12g, Fat: 2g, Carbohydrates: 50g

Butternut Squash and Black Bean Chili

A comforting chili featuring sweet butternut squash, black beans, and warming spices.

Preparation Time: 20 minutes, Cooking Time: 40 minutes, Total Time: 1 hour, serving: 6

Ingredients: 4 cups butternut squash (cubed), 1 can (15 oz) black beans, 1 onion (chopped), 2 cloves garlic (minced), 1 can (14 oz) diced tomatoes, 4 cups vegetable broth, 2 tablespoons chili powder, 1 teaspoon cumin.

Direction:

1. In a large pot, combine butternut squash, black beans, onion, garlic, diced tomatoes, vegetable broth, chili powder, and cumin.
2. Simmer in a low heat for 40 minutes or until squash is tender.
3. Serve hot and enjoy!

Nutritional Info: Calories: 240, Protein: 12g, Fat: 1g, Carbohydrates: 50g

Chickpea and Cauliflower Chili

A hearty chili made with chickpeas, cauliflower, and a blend of spices.

Preparation Time: 15 minutes, Cooking Time: 35 minutes, Total Time: 50 minutes, serving: 6

Ingredients: 2 cups cauliflower florets, 1 can (15 oz) chickpeas, 1 onion (chopped), 2 cloves garlic (minced), 1 can (14 oz) diced tomatoes, 2 cups vegetable broth, 2 tablespoons chili powder, 1 teaspoon cumin.

Direction:

1. In a large pot, sauté onion and garlic until fragrant.
2. Add cauliflower florets, chickpeas, diced tomatoes, vegetable broth, chili powder, and cumin.
3. Simmer over low heat for about 35 minutes and serve hot.

Nutritional Info: Calories: 260, Protein: 14g, Fat: 2g, Carbohydrates: 45g

SANDWICH RECIPES

These sandwiches are not only delicious but also packed with protein, making them perfect for a satisfying and nutritious meal!

Chickpea Salad Sandwich

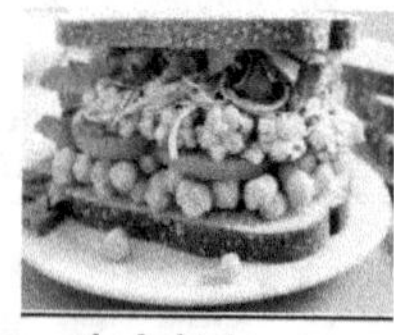

A protein-packed sandwich featuring mashed chickpeas, crunchy vegetables, and creamy avocado.

Preparation Time: 10 minutes, Cooking Time: 0 minutes, Total Time: 10 minutes, serving: 2

Ingredients: 1 can (15 oz) chickpeas (drained and rinsed), 1 ripe avocado (mashed), 1/4 cup diced celery, 1/4 cup diced red onion, 2 tablespoons lemon juice, 1 teaspoon dijon mustard, 4 slices gluten-free bread.

Direction:

1. In a bowl, mash chickpeas and avocado together.
2. Add diced celery, red onion, lemon juice, and dijon mustard, mix well.
3. Spread the mixture onto gluten-free bread slices.
4. Top with another slice of bread to make sandwiches.
5. Cut in half and serve. Enjoy!

Nutritional Info: Calories: 320, Protein: 15g, Fat: 12g, Carbohydrates: 40g

Tofu and Veggie Wrap

A satisfying wrap filled with marinated tofu, crisp vegetables, and hummus.

Preparation Time: 15 minutes, Cooking Time: 10 minutes, Total Time: 25 minutes, serving: 2

Ingredients: 1/2 block (7 oz) extra firm tofu (sliced), 2 gluten-free wraps, 1 cup mixed salad greens, 1/2 cup sliced bell peppers, 1/2 cup shredded carrots, 1/4 cup hummus.

Direction:

1. Marinate tofu slices in your favorite sauce.
2. Sauté in a non-stick pan until golden.
3. Place tofu, salad greens, bell peppers, and shredded carrots on gluten-free wraps.
4. Spread hummus over the fillings. Roll up tightly and slice in half.

Nutritional Info: Calories: 280, Protein: 15g, Fat: 10g, Carbohydrates: 30g

Grilled Portobello Mushroom Sandwich

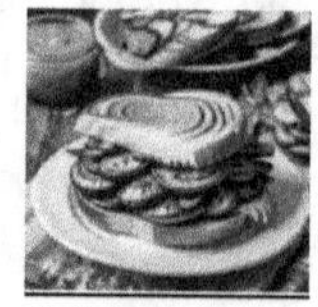

A hearty sandwich featuring grilled portobello mushrooms, roasted red peppers, and creamy avocado.

Preparation Time: 10 minutes, Cooking Time: 10 minutes.Total Time: 20 minutes, srving: 2

Ingredients: 2 large portobello mushrooms, 1/2 cup roasted red peppers, 1 ripe avocado (sliced), 4 slices gluten-free bread, 1 tablespoon balsamic vinegar.

Direction:

1. Marinate portobello mushrooms in balsamic vinegar.
2. Grill or pan-sear until tender. Toast gluten-free bread slices.
3. Layer mushrooms, roasted red peppers, and avocado slices between the bread slices.
4. Serve warm.

Nutritional Info: Calories: 280, Protein: 10g, Fat: 12g, Carbohydrates: 35g

Mashed White Bean and Avocado Wrap

A creamy wrap filled with mashed white beans, avocado, and fresh veggies.

Preparation Time: 10 minutes, Cooking Time: 0 minutes, Total Time: 10 minutes, serving: 2

Ingredients: 1 can (15 oz) white beans (drained and rinsed), 1 ripe avocado (mashed), 2 gluten-free wraps, 1/2 cup sliced cucumber, 1/2 cup shredded lettuce, 1/4 cup diced tomatoes.

Direction:

1. Mash white beans and avocado together in a bowl.
2. Spread the mixture onto gluten-free wraps.
3. Top with sliced cucumber, shredded lettuce, and diced tomatoes.
4. Roll up tightly and slice in half.

Nutritional Info: Calories: 300, Protein: 12g, Fat: 10g, Carbohydrates: 40g

Tempeh Reuben Sandwich

A vegan twist on the classic Reuben sandwich, featuring marinated tempeh, sauerkraut, and dairy-free Thousand Island dressing.

Preparation Time: 15 minutes, Cooking Time: 10 minutes, Total Time: 25 minutes, serving: 2

Ingredients: 1/2 block (7 oz) tempeh (sliced), 4 slices gluten-free bread, 1/2 cup sauerkraut, 1/4 cup dairy-free Thousand Island dressing.

Direction:

1. Marinate tempeh slices in your favorite sauce.
2. Sauté in a non-stick pan until golden.
3. Toast gluten-free bread slices.
4. Spread dairy-free Thousand Island dressing on one side of each slice.

5. Layer tempeh and sauerkraut between the bread slices.
6. Serve warm.
Nutritional Info: Calories: 320, Protein: 14g, Fat: 12g, Carbohydrates: 40g

Pesto Veggie Panini

A flavorful panini filled with homemade pesto, grilled vegetables, and dairy-free cheese.
Preparation Time: 15 minutes, Cooking Time: 10 minutes Total Time: 25 minutes, serving: 2
Ingredients: 4 slices gluten-free bread, 1/4 cup dairy-free pesto, 1/2 cup grilled vegetables (such as zucchini, bell peppers, and eggplant), 1/4 cup dairy-free cheese (shredded).
Direction:
1. Spread dairy-free pesto on two slices of gluten-free bread.
2. Top with grilled vegetables and dairy-free cheese.
3. Place the remaining bread slices
Grilled Tofu and Vegetable Sandwich

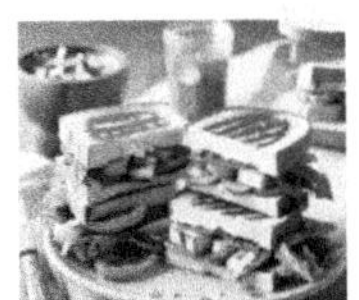

A flavorful sandwich featuring marinated grilled tofu and assorted vegetables.
Preparation Time: 15 minutes, Cooking Time: 10 minutes, Total Time: 25 minutes, Serving: 2
Ingredients: 1/2 block (7 oz) extra firm tofu, 4 slices gluten-free bread, 1/2 cup sliced bell peppers, 1/2 cup sliced zucchini, 1/4 cup sliced red onion, 2 tablespoons balsamic vinegar.
Direction:
1. Marinate tofu slices in balsamic vinegar.
2. Grill tofu along with sliced vegetables until tender.
3. Toast gluten-free bread slices.
4. Assemble sandwiches by placing grilled tofu and vegetables between bread slices.
5. Serve warm and enjoy!
Nutritional Info: Calories: 280, Protein: 14g, Fat: 8g, Carbohydrates: 38g

Avocado and Hummus Wrap

A creamy and satisfying wrap filled with mashed avocado, hummus, and crunchy vegetables.
Preparation Time: 10 minutes, Cooking Time: 0 minutes, Total Time: 10 minutes, serving: 2
Ingredients: 2 gluten-free wraps, 1 avocado, 1/4 cup hummus, 1/2 cup shredded carrots, 1/2 cup shredded lettuce, 1/4 cup sliced cucumber.
Direction:
1. Mash avocado and spread it onto gluten-free wraps.
2. Spread hummus over the avocado layer.
3. Top with shredded carrots, lettuce, and sliced cucumber.

4. Roll up the wraps tightly and slice in half.
5. Serve fresh. Enjoy!
Nutritional Info: Calories: 300, Protein: 8g, Fat: 16g, Carbohydrates: 35g

Tempeh Bacon BLT Sandwich

A plant-based twist on the classic BLT sandwich featuring crispy tempeh bacon, lettuce, and tomato.

Preparation Time: 10 minutes, Cooking Time: 10 minutes, Total Time: 20 minutes, serving: 2

Ingredients: 1/2 block (7 oz) tempeh, 4 slices gluten-free bread, 1 tomato (sliced), 1 cup shredded lettuce, 2 tablespoons maple syrup, 1 tablespoon soy sauce.

Direction:
1. Slice tempeh thinly.
2. Mix maple syrup and soy sauce to make a marinade.
3. Marinate tempeh slices in the mixture.
4. Pan-fry tempeh until crispy.
5. Toast gluten-free bread slices.
6. Assemble sandwiches with tempeh bacon, lettuce, and tomato.
7. Serve warm.
Nutritional Info: Calories: 280, Protein: 16g, Fat: 6g, Carbohydrates: 40g

Mushroom and Eggplant Panini

A hearty and flavorful panini featuring grilled mushrooms, eggplant, and dairy-free cheese.
Preparation Time: 15 minutes, Cooking Time: 10 minutes, Total Time: 25 minutes, serving: 2

Ingredients: 4 slices gluten-free bread, 1 cup sliced mushrooms, 1 cup sliced eggplant, 1/4 cup dairy-free cheese shreds, 2 tablespoons balsamic vinegar.

Direction:
1. Marinate mushrooms and eggplant in balsamic vinegar.
2. Grill or pan-sear until tender. Toast gluten-free bread slices.
3. Assemble sandwiches with grilled mushrooms, eggplant, and dairy-free cheese.
4. Grill in a panini press until cheese melts. Serve hot.
Nutritional Info: Calories: 260, Protein: 10g, Fat: 8g, Carbohydrates: 40g

Peanut Butter and Banana Sandwich

A classic and simple sandwich made with creamy peanut butter and sliced banana.
Preparation Time: 5 minutes, Cooking Time: 0 minutes, Total Time: 5 minutes, serving: 2
Ingredients: 4 slices gluten-free bread, 1/2 cup peanut butter, 1 banana (sliced).

Direction:
1. Spread peanut butter evenly on gluten-free bread slices.
2. Top with sliced banana and another slice of bread to make sandwiches.
3. Slice in half and serve fresh.
Nutritional Info: Calories: 320, Protein: 10g, Fat: 16g, Carbohydrates: 40g

Hummus and Roasted Vegetable Sandwich

A flavorful sandwich featuring roasted vegetables and creamy hummus.
Preparation Time: 15 minutes, Cooking Time: 20 minutes, Total Time: 35 minutes, serving: 2
Ingredients: 4 slices gluten-free bread, 1/2 cup hummus, 1 cup mixed roasted vegetables (such as bell peppers, zucchini, and onions).
Direction:
1. Roast mixed vegetables until tender.
2. Toast gluten-free bread slices.
3. Spread hummus on each slice.
4. Top with roasted vegetables and another slice of bread.
5. Serve warm.
Nutritional Info: Calories: 280, Protein: 10g, Fat: 10g, Carbohydrates: 38g

Tofu Banh Mi Sandwich

A Vietnamese-inspired sandwich featuring marinated tofu, pickled vegetables, and fresh herbs.
Preparation Time: 20 minutes, Cooking Time: 10 minutes, Total Time: 30 minutes, serving: 2
Ingredients: 1/2 block (7 oz) extra firm tofu, 4 slices gluten-free bread, 1/4 cup pickled vegetables (carrots, daikon radish), 1/4 cup sliced cucumber, 1/4 cup fresh cilantro leaves, 2 tablespoons soy sauce, 1 tablespoon rice vinegar.
Direction:
1. Marinate tofu slices in soy sauce.
2. Pan-fry until golden.
3. Toast gluten-free bread slices.
4. Assemble sandwiches with tofu, pickled vegetables, sliced cucumber, and cilantro.
5. Serve fresh.
Nutritional Info: Calories: 280, Protein: 14g, Fat: 8g, Carbohydrates: 38g

Quinoa and Roasted Red Pepper Wrap

A nutritious wrap filled with quinoa, roasted red peppers, and creamy avocado.
Preparation Time: 15 minutes, Cooking Time: 20 minutes, Total Time: 35 minutes, serving: 2
Ingredients: 2 gluten-free wraps, 1 cup cooked quinoa, 1/2 cup roasted red peppers, 1 avocado (sliced), 1/4 cup hummus.
Direction:
1. Cook quinoa according to package instructions.
2. Warm gluten-free wraps.
3. Spread hummus on each wrap.
4. Top with cooked quinoa, roasted red peppers, avocado slices, and roll tightly.
5. Slice in half and serve.
Nutritional Info: Calories: 320, Protein: 10g, Fat: 16g, Carbohydrates: 40g

Eggplant and Tomato Sandwich

A simple yet flavorful sandwich featuring grilled eggplant, fresh tomatoes, and basil.

Preparation Time: 10 minutes, Cooking Time: 10 minutes, Total Time: 20 minutes, serving: 2
Ingredients: 4 slices gluten-free bread, 1 small eggplant (sliced), 1 large tomato (sliced), 1/4 cup fresh basil leaves.
Direction:
1. Grill or pan-sear eggplant slices until tender.
2. Toast gluten-free bread slices.
3. Layer grilled eggplant, tomato slices, and fresh basil leaves between bread slices.
4. Serve warm.
Nutritional Info: Calories: 260, Protein: 8g, Fat: 8g, Carbohydrates: 38g

BURGER RECIPES

Chickpea Spinach Burgers

These hearty burgers combine chickpeas and spinach for a nutritious and flavorful meal.
Preparation Time: 15 minutes, Cooking Time: 20 minutes, Total Time: 35 minutes, serving: 4
Ingredients: 1 can chickpeas, drained and rinsed, 2 cups fresh spinach, chopped, 1/4 cup gluten-free rolled oats, 1/4 cup finely chopped onion, 2 cloves garlic, minced, 2 tablespoons ground flaxseed mixed with 6 tablespoons water (flax egg substitute), 1 teaspoon smoked paprika
Directions:
1. In a food processor, pulse chickpeas until coarsely mashed.
2. Transfer to a bowl and add chopped spinach, rolled oats, onion, minced garlic, flax egg substitute, and smoked paprika.
4. Mix until well combined. Form the mixture into patties. Cook in a skillet over medium heat for 8-10 minutes on each side until golden brown.
5. Serve on lettuce wraps or gluten-free buns with your favorite toppings.
Nutritional Info: Calories: 220, Protein: 10g, Fat: 5g, Carbohydrates: 35g

Lentil Mushroom Burgers

These savory burgers feature lentils and mushrooms, packed with protein and flavor.
Preparation Time: 20 minutes, Cooking Time: 25 minutes, Total Time: 45 minutes, serving: 4
Ingredients: 1 cup cooked lentils, 1 cup finely chopped mushrooms, 1/4 cup gluten-free breadcrumbs, 1/4 cup finely chopped onion, 2 cloves garlic, minced, 2 tablespoons ground flaxseed mixed with 6 tablespoons water (flax egg substitute), 1 teaspoon dried thyme
Directions:
1. In a skillet, sauté mushrooms until tender.
2. In a large bowl, mash cooked lentils and add sautéed mushrooms, breadcrumbs, onion, garlic, flax egg substitute, and dried thyme. Mix until well combined.
3. Form the mixture into patties.
4. Cook in a skillet over medium heat for 8-10 minutes on each side until crispy.

5. Serve on gluten-free buns with avocado slices and tomato.
Nutritional Info: Calories: 250, Protein: 12g, Fat: 6g, Carbohydrates: 40g

Black Bean Quinoa Burgers

These protein-packed burgers are made with black beans, quinoa, and flavorful spices.
Preparation Time: 15 minutes, Cooking Time: 20 minutes, Total Time: 35 minutes, serving: 4
Ingredients: 1 can black beans, drained and rinsed, 1 cup cooked quinoa, 1/4 cup gluten-free breadcrumbs, 1/4 cup finely chopped onion, 2 cloves garlic, minced, 2 tablespoons ground flaxseed mixed with 6 tablespoons water (flax egg substitute), 1 teaspoon chili powder
Directions:
1. In a medium mixing bowl, mash black beans with a fork.
2. Add cooked quinoa, breadcrumbs, onion, garlic, flax egg substitute, and chili powder. Mix until well combined. Form the mixture into patties.
3. Cook in a skillet over medium heat for 8-10 minutes on each side until golden brown.
4. Serve on lettuce wraps or gluten-free buns with salsa and guacamole.
Nutritional Info: Calories: 240, Protein: 11g, Fat: 5g, Carbohydrates: 38g

Lentil Sweet Potato Burgers

These wholesome burgers feature lentils, sweet potatoes, and aromatic spices for a delicious meal.
Preparation Time: 20 minutes, Cooking Time: 25 minutes, Total Time: 45 minutes, serving: 4
Ingredients: 1 cup cooked lentils, 1 cup mashed sweet potato, 1/4 cup gluten-free oats, 1/4 cup finely chopped onion, 2 cloves garlic, minced, 2 tablespoons ground flaxseed mixed with 6 tablespoons water (flax egg substitute), 1 teaspoon smoked paprika
Directions:
1. In a bowl, mash cooked lentils and mix with mashed sweet potato, oats, onion, garlic, flax egg substitute, and smoked paprika.
2. Form the mixture into patties.
3. Cook in a skillet over medium heat for 8-10 minutes on each side until crispy.
4. Serve on lettuce wraps or gluten-free buns with avocado slices and arugula.
Nutritional Info: Calories: 230, Protein: 10g, Fat: 4g, Carbohydrates: 38g

Portobello Mushroom Burgers

Juicy portobello mushrooms marinated in balsamic vinegar and herbs, served with fresh lettuce and tomato.
Preparation Time: 10 minutes, Cooking Time: 15 minutes, Total Time: 25 minutes, serving: 4
Ingredients: 4 large portobello mushrooms, 2 tablespoons olive oil (optional), 1/4 cup balsamic vinegar, 2 cloves garlic, minced, 1 teaspoon dried thyme
Directions:

1. In a shallow dish, whisk together balsamic vinegar, olive oil (if using), minced garlic, and dried thyme. 2. Place portobello mushrooms in the marinade, turning to coat.
3. Let marinate for 10 minutes.
4. Heat a grill or grill pan over medium heat.
5. Cook mushrooms for 5-7 minutes on each side until tender.
6. Serve on gluten-free buns with lettuce and tomato.
Nutritional Info: Calories: 120, Protein: 5g, Fat: 3g, Carbohydrates: 20g

Tofu Veggie Burgers

Flavorful tofu burgers loaded with vegetables and spices, perfect for a plant-based meal.

Preparation Time: 20 minutes, Cooking Time: 20 minutes, Total Time: 40 minutes, serving: 4

Ingredients: 1 block tofu, pressed and crumbled, 1 cup shredded carrots, 1/2 cup finely chopped bell pepper, 1/4 cup gluten-free breadcrumbs, 2 tablespoons nutritional yeast, 2 tablespoons ground flaxseed mixed with 6 tablespoons water (flax egg substitute), 1 teaspoon smoked paprika

Directions:

1. In a large bowl, mix crumbled tofu, shredded carrots, chopped bell pepper, breadcrumbs, nutritional yeast, flax egg substitute, and smoked paprika.
2. Form the mixture into patties.
3. Cook in a skillet over medium heat for 8-10 minutes on each side until golden brown.
4. Serve on lettuce wraps or gluten-free buns with avocado slices and sprouts.
Nutritional Info: Calories: 210, Protein: 9g, Fat: 5g, Carbohydrates: 30g

Cauliflower Chickpea Burgers

These flavorful burgers feature cauliflower and chickpeas, seasoned with spices and herbs for a satisfying meal.

Preparation Time: 25 minutes, Cooking Time: 20 minutes, Total Time: 45 minutes, serving: 4

Ingredients: 2 cups cauliflower florets, 1 can chickpeas, drained and rinsed, 1/4 cup gluten-free breadcrumbs, 1/4 cup finely chopped onion, 2 cloves garlic, minced, 2 tablespoons ground flaxseed mixed with 6 tablespoons water (flax egg substitute), 1 teaspoon curry powder

Directions:

1. Steam cauliflower florets until tender.
2. In a food processor, pulse steamed cauliflower and chickpeas until finely chopped.
3. Transfer to a bowl and add breadcrumbs, onion, garlic, flax egg substitute, and curry powder.
4. Mix until well combined and then form the mixture into patties.
5. Cook in a skillet over medium heat for 8-10 minutes on each side until crispy.
6. Serve on lettuce wraps or gluten-free buns with sliced cucumber and tahini sauce.
Nutritional Info: Calories: 220, Protein: 10g, Fat: 5g, Carbohydrates: 35g

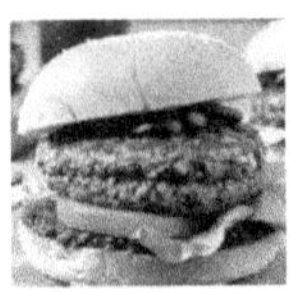

Black Bean and Quinoa Burger

A hearty burger made with black beans, quinoa, and flavorful spices.

Preparation Time: 15 minutes, Cooking Time: 20 minutes, Total Time: 35 minutes, serving: 4

Ingredients: 1 can (15 oz) black beans (drained and rinsed), 1 cup cooked quinoa, 1/4 cup diced onion, 1/4 cup chopped cilantro, 1 teaspoon cumin, 1/2 teaspoon paprika, 4 gluten-free burger buns.

Direction:

1. In a bowl, mash black beans.
2. Add cooked quinoa, diced onion, chopped cilantro, cumin, and paprika.
3. Mix until well combined. Form mixture into patties and grill or bake until cooked through.
4. Serve on gluten-free burger buns.

Nutritional Info: Calories: 220, Protein: 10g, Fat: 2g, Carbohydrates: 40g

Lentil and Mushroom Burger

A savory burger made with lentils, mushrooms, and aromatic herbs.

Preparation Time: 20 minutes, Cooking Time: 25 minutes, Total Time: 45 minutes, serving: 4

Ingredients: 1 cup cooked lentils, 1 cup chopped mushrooms, 1/4 cup diced onion, 2 cloves garlic (minced), 1 tablespoon chopped parsley, 1 teaspoon dried thyme, 4 gluten-free burger buns.

Direction:

1. In a skillet, sauté mushrooms, onion, and garlic until softened.
2. In a bowl, mash cooked lentils and mix with sautéed vegetables, parsley, and thyme.
3. Form mixture into patties and cook on a skillet until golden brown.
4. Serve on gluten-free burger buns.

Nutritional Info: Calories: 200, Protein: 12g, Fat: 3g, Carbohydrates: 35g

Chickpea and Spinach Burger

A nutritious burger made with chickpeas, spinach, and aromatic spices.

Preparation Time: 15 minutes, Cooking Time: 20 minutes, Total Time: 35 minutes, serving: 4

Ingredients: 1 can (15 oz) chickpeas (drained and rinsed), 1 cup chopped spinach, 1/4 cup diced red bell pepper, 1/4 cup diced onion, 1 teaspoon cumin, 1/2 teaspoon smoked paprika, 4 gluten-free burger buns.

Direction:

1. In a food processor, pulse chickpeas until coarsely mashed.

2. Transfer to a bowl and mix in chopped spinach, red bell pepper, onion, cumin, and smoked paprika.
3. Form mixture into patties and grill or bake until firm.
4. Serve on gluten-free burger buns.
Nutritional Info: Calories: 230, Protein: 9g, Fat: 3g, Carbohydrates: 40g

Sweet Potato and Black Bean Burger

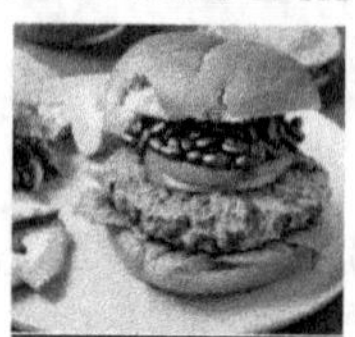

A flavorful burger made with mashed sweet potatoes, black beans, and aromatic spices.
Preparation Time: 25 minutes, Cooking Time: 30 minutes, Total Time: 55 minutes, serving: 4
Ingredients: 2 cups mashed sweet potatoes, 1 can (15 oz) black beans (drained and rinsed), 1/4 cup diced red onion, 1/4 cup chopped cilantro, 1 teaspoon chili powder, 1/2 teaspoon cumin, 4 gluten-free burger buns.
Direction
1. In a bowl, mash cooked sweet potatoes and black beans together.
2. Mix in diced red onion, chopped cilantro, chili powder, and cumin.
3. Form mixture into patties and grill or bake until cooked through.
4. Serve on gluten-free burger buns.
Nutritional Info: Calories: 240, Protein: 10g, Fat: 2g, Carbohydrates: 45g

Soy and Walnut Burger

A protein-rich burger made with soy granules, walnuts, and aromatic herbs.
Preparation Time: 20 minutes, Cooking Time: 25 minutes, Total Time: 45 minutes, serving: 4
Ingredients: 1 cup soy granules, 1/2 cup chopped walnuts, 1/4 cup diced onion, 2 cloves garlic (minced), 1 tablespoon chopped parsley, 1 teaspoon dried oregano, 4 gluten-free burger buns.
Direction:
1. In a bowl, soak soy granules in water for 10 minutes, then drain.
2. In a food processor, pulse soaked soy granules and walnuts until coarse.
3. Transfer to a bowl and mix in diced onion, minced garlic, parsley, and oregano.
4. Form mixture into patties and cook on a skillet until golden.
5. Serve on gluten-free burger buns.
Nutritional Info: Calories: 220, Protein: 15g, Fat: 6g, Carbohydrates: 30g

Edamame and Brown Rice Burger

A wholesome burger made with edamame, brown rice, and aromatic spices.
Preparation Time: 25 minutes, Cooking Time: 30 minutes, Total Time: 55 minutes, serving: 4

Ingredients: 1 cup cooked edamame, 1 cup cooked brown rice, 1/4 cup diced red bell pepper, 1/4 cup diced onion, 1 tablespoon chopped cilantro, 1 teaspoon ground coriander, 4 gluten-free burger buns.

Direction:

1. In a bowl, mash cooked edamame and brown rice together.
2. Mix in diced red bell pepper, onion, cilantro, and ground coriander.
3. Form mixture into patties and grill or bake until firm.
4. Serve on gluten-free burger buns.

Nutritional Info: Calories: 230, Protein: 11g, Fat: 3g, Carbohydrates: 40g

Tofu and Sunflower Seed Burger

A protein-packed burger made with tofu, sunflower seeds, and aromatic seasonings.

Preparation Time: 20 minutes, Cooking Time: 25 minutes, Total Time: 45 minutes, serving: 4

Ingredients: 1/2 block (7 oz) extra firm tofu, 1/2 cup sunflower seeds, 1/4 cup diced onion, 2 cloves garlic (minced), 1 tablespoon nutritional yeast, 1 teaspoon dried basil, 4 gluten-free burger buns.

Direction:

1. In a food processor, pulse tofu and sunflower seeds until course.
2. Transfer to a bowl and mix in diced onion, minced garlic, nutritional yeast, and dried basil.
3. Form mixture into patties and cook on a skillet until golden.
4. Serve on gluten-free burger buns.

Nutritional Info: Calories: 240, Protein: 14g, Fat: 8g, Carbohydrates: 30g

Chia Seed and Chickpea Burger

A nutritious burger made with chia seeds, chickpeas, and flavorful spices.

Preparation Time: 15 minutes, Cooking Time: 20 minutes, Total Time: 35 minutes, serving: 4

Ingredients: 1/4 cup chia seeds, 1 can (15 oz) chickpeas (drained and rinsed), 1/4 cup diced red onion, 1/4 cup chopped parsley, 1 teaspoon smoked paprika, 1/2 teaspoon ground cumin, 4 gluten-free burger buns.

Direction:

1. In a bowl, soak chia seeds in water for 10 minutes.
2. In a food processor, pulse chickpeas until coarsely mashed.
3. Transfer to a bowl and mix in soaked chia seeds, diced red onion, chopped parsley, smoked paprika, and ground cumin.
4. Form mixture into patties and grill or bake until cooked through.
5. Serve on gluten-free burger buns.

Nutritional Info: Calories: 230, Protein: 12g, Fat: 5g, Carbohydrates: 35g

Mushroom and Lentil Burger

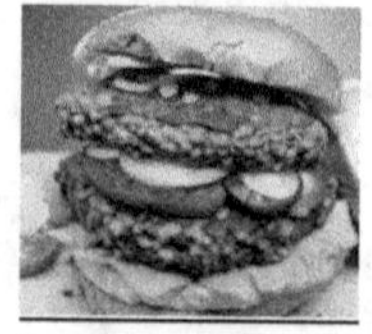

A savory burger made with hearty mushrooms, lentils, and aromatic seasonings.
Preparation Time: 20 minutes, Cooking Time: 25 minutes, Total Time: 45 minutes, serving: 4

Ingredients: 1 cup cooked lentils, 1 cup chopped mushrooms, 1/4 cup diced onion, 2 cloves garlic (minced), 1 tablespoon soy sauce, 1 teaspoon dried thyme, 4 gluten-free burger buns.

Direction:
1. In a skillet, sauté mushrooms, onion, and garlic until softened.
2. In a bowl, mash cooked lentils and mix with sautéed vegetables, soy sauce, and dried thyme.
3. Form mixture into patties and cook on a skillet until golden.
4. Serve on gluten-free burger buns.
Nutritional Info: Calories: 220, Protein: 11g, Fat: 3g, Carbohydrates: 35g

Sweet Potato and Chickpea Burger

A delicious burger made with mashed sweet potatoes, chickpeas, and aromatic spices.
Preparation Time: 25 minutes, Cooking Time: 30 minutes, Total Time: 55 minutes, serving: 4

Ingredients: 2 cups mashed sweet potatoes, 1 can (15 oz) chickpeas (drained and rinsed), 1/4 cup diced red onion, 1/4 cup chopped cilantro, 1 teaspoon ground cumin, 1/2 teaspoon smoked paprika, 4 gluten-free burger buns.

Direction:
1. In a bowl, mash cooked sweet potatoes and chickpeas together.
2. Mix in diced red onion, chopped cilantro, ground cumin, and smoked paprika.
3. Form mixture into patties and grill or bake until firm.
4. Serve on gluten-free burger buns.
Nutritional Info: Calories: 240, Protein: 10g, Fat: 3g, Carbohydrates: 40g

PIZZA RECIPES

Chickpea Crust Pizza

A protein-rich pizza crust made with chickpea flour topped with colorful vegetables.
Preparation Time: 15 minutes, Cooking Time: 25 minutes, Total Time: 40 minutes, serving: 2

Ingredients: 1 cup chickpea flour, 1/2 cup water, 1/2 teaspoon baking powder, 1/4 cup tomato sauce, 1/4 cup sliced bell peppers, 1/4 cup sliced mushrooms, 1/4 cup chopped spinach.

Direction:

1. Preheat oven to 400°F (200°C). Mix chickpea flour, water, and baking powder to form a dough.
2. Spread dough onto a baking sheet.
3. Top with tomato sauce, bell peppers, mushrooms, and spinach.
4. Bake for 25 minutes or until crust is crispy.
5. Slice and serve.

Nutritional Info: Calories: 280, Protein: 14g, Fat: 4g, Carbohydrates: 45g

Cauliflower Crust Pizza

A low-carb pizza crust made with cauliflower, topped with dairy-free cheese and fresh herbs.

Preparation Time: 20 minutes, Cooking Time: 30 minutes, Total Time: 50 minutes, serving: 2

Ingredients: 1 cauliflower head (riced), 1/2 cup almond flour, 1 flax egg (1 tablespoon ground flaxseed + 3 tablespoons water), 1/4 cup tomato sauce, 1/2 cup dairy-free cheese, 1/4 cup sliced olives, 1/4 cup chopped basil.

Direction:

1. Preheat oven to 425°F (220°C).
2. Mix cauliflower rice, almond flour, and flax egg to form a dough.
3. Press dough onto a baking sheet. Bake for 25 minutes or until crust is golden brown.
4. Top with tomato sauce, dairy-free cheese, olives, and basil.
5. Bake for another 5 minutes.
6. Slice and serve.

Nutritional Info: Calories: 240, Protein: 12g, Fat: 6g, Carbohydrates: 35g

Quinoa Crust Pizza

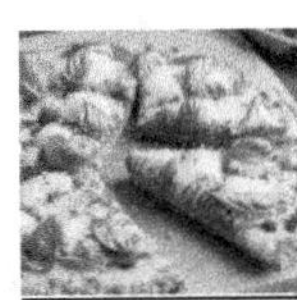

A nutritious pizza crust made with quinoa flour topped with plant-based ingredients.

Preparation Time: 20 minutes, Cooking Time: 30 minutes, Total Time: 50 minutes, serving: 2

Ingredients: 1 cup quinoa flour, 1/2 cup water, 1/2 teaspoon baking powder, 1/4 cup marinara sauce, 1/4 cup sliced cherry tomatoes, 1/4 cup chopped bell peppers, 1/4 cup chopped kale.

Direction:

1. Preheat oven to 400°F (200°C).
2. Mix quinoa flour, water, and baking powder to form a dough.
3. Spread dough onto a baking sheet.
4. Top with marinara sauce, cherry tomatoes, bell peppers, and kale.
5. Bake for 30 minutes or until crust is crispy.
6. Slice and serve.

Nutritional Info: Calories: 250, Protein: 12g, Fat: 5g, Carbohydrates: 40g

Sweet Potato Crust Pizza

A flavorful pizza crust made with mashed sweet potatoes, topped with dairy-free cheese and roasted vegetables.

Preparation Time: 25 minutes, Cooking Time: 35 minutes, Total Time: 60 minutes, serving: 2

Ingredients: 1 large sweet potato (cooked and mashed), 1/2 cup chickpea flour, 1/4 cup water, 1/2 teaspoon baking powder, 1/4 cup tomato sauce, 1/2 cup dairy-free cheese, 1/4 cup sliced bell peppers, 1/4 cup sliced mushrooms.

Direction:

1. Preheat oven to 425°F (220°C).
2. Mix mashed sweet potato, chickpea flour, water, and baking powder to form a dough.
3. Press dough onto a baking sheet. Bake for 25 minutes.
4. Top with tomato sauce, dairy-free cheese, bell peppers, and mushrooms.
5. Bake for another 10 minutes.
6. Slice and serve.

Nutritional Info: Calories: 270, Protein: 14g, Fat: 4g, Carbohydrates: 45g

Zucchini Crust Pizza

A light and crispy pizza crust made with shredded zucchini, topped with dairy-free cheese and fresh vegetables.

Preparation Time: 15 minutes, Cooking Time: 25 minutes, Total Time: 40 minutes, serving: 2

Ingredients: 2 cups shredded zucchini, 1/2 cup almond flour, 1/4 cup water, 1/2 teaspoon baking powder, 1/4 cup tomato sauce, 1/2 cup dairy-free cheese, 1/4 cup sliced cherry tomatoes, 1/4 cup chopped basil.

Direction:

1. Preheat oven to 425°F (220°C).
2. Mix shredded zucchini, almond flour, water, and baking powder to form a dough.
3. Press dough onto a baking sheet. Bake for 20 minutes.
4. Top with tomato sauce, dairy-free cheese, cherry tomatoes, and basil.
5. Bake for another 5 minutes.
6. Slice and serve.

Nutritional Info: Calories: 240, Protein: 12g, Fat: 6g, Carbohydrates: 35g

Spinach and Mushroom Pizza

A delicious pizza topped with dairy-free spinach sauce, mushrooms, and cherry tomatoes.

Preparation Time: 20 minutes, Cooking Time: 30 minutes, Total Time: 50 minutes, serving: 2

Ingredients: 1 cup packed spinach, 1/4 cup almond milk, 1 tablespoon nutritional yeast, 1/4 teaspoon garlic powder, 1/4 cup sliced mushrooms, 1/4 cup sliced cherry tomatoes, 1/4 cup sliced black olives.

Direction:

1. Preheat oven to 425°F (220°C).

2. In a blender, blend spinach, almond milk, nutritional yeast, and garlic powder to make the sauce.
3. Spread sauce onto a pizza crust.
4. Top with mushrooms, cherry tomatoes, and black olives.
5. Bake for 25 minutes or until toppings are cooked.
6. Slice and serve.
Nutritional Info: Calories: 230, Protein: 10g, Fat: 6g, Carbohydrates: 35g

Mediterranean Chickpea Pizza

A flavorful pizza topped with a creamy chickpea spread, olives, and roasted red peppers.
Preparation Time: 25 minutes, Cooking Time: 30 minutes, Total Time: 55 minutes, serving: 2
Ingredients: 1 can (15 oz) chickpeas (drained and rinsed), 2 tablespoons tahini, 2 tablespoons lemon juice, 1 clove garlic (minced), 1/4 cup sliced kalamata olives, 1/4 cup chopped roasted red peppers.
Direction:
1. Preheat oven to 425°F (220°C).
2. In a food processor, blend chickpeas, tahini, lemon juice, and garlic until smooth.
3. Spread the chickpea mixture onto a pizza crust.
4. Top with olives and roasted red peppers.
5. Bake for 25 minutes or until crust is crispy.
6. Slice and serve.
Nutritional Info: Calories: 250, Protein: 12g, Fat: 7g, Carbohydrates: 35g

Thai Peanut Pizza

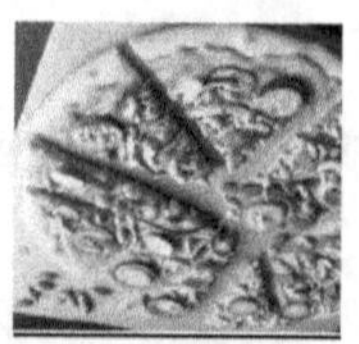

A unique pizza topped with a creamy peanut sauce, tofu, and fresh vegetables.
Preparation Time: 20 minutes, Cooking Time: 25 minutes, Total Time: 45 minutes, serving: 2
Ingredients: 1/4 cup peanut butter, 2 tablespoons soy sauce, 1 tablespoon maple syrup, 1 tablespoon lime juice, 1/4 teaspoon ginger powder, 1/4 cup cubed tofu, 1/4 cup sliced red bell peppers, 1/4 cup sliced green onions.
Direction:
1. Preheat oven to 425°F (220°C).
2. In a bowl, whisk together peanut butter, soy sauce, maple syrup, lime juice, and ginger powder to make the sauce.
3. Spread the sauce onto a pizza crust.
4. Top with tofu, red bell peppers, and green onions.
5. Bake for 20 minutes or until toppings are cooked.
6. Slice and serve.
Nutritional Info: Calories: 260, Protein: 13g, Fat: 8g, Carbohydrates: 35g

Black Bean and Corn Pizza

A Tex-Mex inspired pizza topped with black beans, corn, avocado, and salsa.
Preparation Time: 20 minutes, Cooking Time: 25 minutes, Total Time: 45 minutes, serving: 2
Ingredients: 1/2 cup canned black beans (drained and rinsed), 1/2 cup corn kernels, 1/4 cup diced red onion, 1/4 cup chopped cilantro, 1/4 cup salsa, 1/2 avocado (sliced).
Direction:
1. Preheat oven to 425°F (220°C).
2. Spread black beans and corn onto a pizza crust.
3. Top with diced red onion and chopped cilantro. Bake for 20 minutes.
4. Remove from oven and top with salsa and sliced avocado.
5. Slice and serve.
Nutritional Info: Calories: 270, Protein: 12g, Fat: 8g, Carbohydrates: 40g

Mushroom and Arugula Pizza

A gourmet-style pizza topped with sautéed mushrooms, arugula, and dairy-free cheese.
Preparation Time: 25 minutes, Cooking Time: 30 minutes, Total Time: 55 minutes, serving: 2
Ingredients: 1 cup sliced mushrooms, 2 cups arugula, 1/4 cup sliced red onion, 1/4 cup dairy-free cheese, 1 tablespoon balsamic glaze.
Direction:
1. Preheat oven to 425°F (220°C). Sauté sliced mushrooms in a skillet until tender.

2. Spread mushrooms onto a pizza crust.
3. Top with arugula, red onion, and dairy-free cheese.
4. Bake for 25 minutes or until cheese is melted.
5. Drizzle with balsamic glaze before serving.
6. Slice and serve.
Nutritional Info: Calories: 260, Protein: 11g, Fat: 6g, Carbohydrates: 40g

NOODLE RECIPES

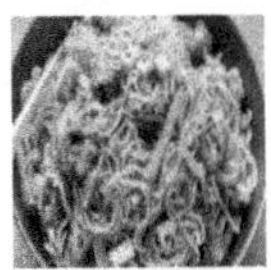

Quinoa Noodle Stir-Fry

A nutritious stir-fry featuring gluten-free quinoa noodles with colorful vegetables and tofu for added protein.

Preparation Time: 15 minutes, Cooking Time: 10 minutes, Total Time: 25 minutes, serving: 4

Ingredients: 8 oz gluten-free quinoa noodles, 1 cup mixed vegetables (bell peppers, broccoli, carrots), 1/2 cup tofu, cubed, 2 tablespoons coconut aminos, 1 tablespoon sesame oil, 1 tablespoon rice vinegar, 1 teaspoon grated ginger, 1 clove garlic, minced

Directions:
1. Cook quinoa noodles according to package instructions.
2. In a pan, sauté mixed vegetables and tofu until vegetables are tender.
3. Add coconut aminos, sesame oil, rice vinegar, ginger, and garlic. Stir well.
4. Add cooked noodles and toss until heated through. Serve hot.
Nutritional Info: Calories: 250, Protein: 12g, Fat: 6g, Carbohydrates: 40g

Chickpea Pasta with Spinach Pesto

Chickpea pasta served with a vibrant spinach pesto, bursting with flavor and protein.

Preparation Time: 15 minutes, Cooking Time: 10 minutes, Total Time: 25 minutes, serving: 4

Ingredients: 8 oz gluten-free chickpea pasta, 2 cups fresh spinach, 1/4 cup pine nuts, 2 tablespoons nutritional yeast, 2 tablespoons lemon juice, 2 cloves garlic, 1/4 cup olive oil

Directions:
1. Cook chickpea pasta according to package instructions.
2. In a food processor, combine spinach, pine nuts, nutritional yeast, lemon juice, garlic, and olive oil.
3. Blend until smooth to make the pesto sauce.
4. Toss cooked pasta with spinach pesto until well coated. Serve warm.

Nutritional Info: Calories: 290, Protein: 14g, Fat: 10g, Carbohydrates: 35g

Tofu Pad Thai

Classic Pad Thai made with rice noodles and tofu, tossed in a flavorful sauce for a protein-rich meal.

Preparation Time: 20 minutes, Cooking Time: 15 minutes, Total Time: 35 minutes, serving: 4

Ingredients: 8 oz rice noodles, 1/2 cup tofu, diced, 1 cup bean sprouts, 1/2 cup shredded carrots, 1/4 cup chopped peanuts, 2 tablespoons tamarind paste, 2 tablespoons coconut aminos, 1 tablespoon maple syrup, 1 tablespoon lime juice, 2 cloves garlic, minced

Directions:

1. Cook rice noodles according to package instructions.
2. In a wok or large skillet, sauté tofu, bean sprouts, shredded carrots, and minced garlic until tofu is golden brown.
3. Add cooked noodles, tamarind paste, coconut aminos, maple syrup, and lime juice. Stir well to combine.
4. Garnished with chopped peanuts and Serve hot.

Nutritional Info: Calories: 320, Protein: 15g, Fat: 10g, Carbohydrates: 45g

Spaghetti Squash Noodles with Lentil Bolognese

Tender spaghetti squash noodles topped with a hearty lentil Bolognese sauce, a nutritious twist on a classic dish.

Preparation Time: 20 minutes, Cooking Time: 45 minutes, Total Time: 65 minutes, serving: 4

Ingredients: 1 medium spaghetti squash, 1 cup cooked lentils, 1 can crushed tomatoes, 1 onion, diced, 2 cloves garlic, minced, 1 teaspoon dried basil, 1 teaspoon dried oregano, 1/4 cup nutritional yeast

Directions:

1. Preheat the oven to 400°F (200°C).
2. Cut the spaghetti squash in half lengthwise and scoop out the seeds.
3. Place the squash halves cut side down on a baking sheet and bake for 40-45 minutes or until tender.
4. In a skillet, sauté onion and garlic until softened.
5. Add cooked lentils, crushed tomatoes, dried basil, and dried oregano and let it simmer for 10 minutes on low heat.
6. Use a fork to scrape the spaghetti squash into noodles.
7. To serve topped with lentil Bolognese sauce and nutritional yeast. Enjoy!

Nutritional Info: Calories: 250, Protein: 12g, Fat: 5g, Carbohydrates: 40g

Thai Peanut Zucchini Noodles

Spiralized zucchini noodles coated in a creamy Thai peanut sauce, topped with tofu for added protein.

Preparation Time: 15 minutes, Cooking Time: 10 minutes, Total Time: 25 minutes, serving: 4

Ingredients: 4 medium zucchinis, spiralized, 1/2 cup tofu, diced, 1/4 cup peanut butter, 2 tablespoons coconut aminos, 1 tablespoon lime juice, 1 tablespoon maple syrup, 1 clove garlic, minced

Directions:

1. In a small bowl, whisk together peanut butter, coconut aminos, lime juice, maple syrup, and minced garlic to make the sauce.
2. In a skillet, sauté diced tofu until golden brown.
3. Add spiralized zucchini noodles and sauce to the skillet.
4. Cook for 2-3 minutes until noodles are tender and coated in sauce. Serve hot and enjoy!

Nutritional Info: Calories: 270, Protein: 14g, Fat: 10g, Carbohydrates: 35g

Mushroom Spinach Pasta

A comforting pasta dish with gluten-free noodles, sautéed mushrooms, and spinach, packed with protein and flavor.

Preparation Time: 15 minutes, Cooking Time: 20 minutes, Total Time: 35 minutes, serving: 4

Ingredients: 8 oz gluten-free pasta, 2 cups sliced mushrooms, 2 cups fresh spinach, 2 cloves garlic, minced, 1/4 cup vegetable broth, 2 tablespoons nutritional yeast, 1 tablespoon olive oil (optional)

Directions:

1. Cook gluten-free pasta according to package instructions.
2. In a large skillet, sauté sliced mushrooms and minced garlic in olive oil (if using) until mushrooms are tender.
3. Add fresh spinach and vegetable broth and cook until spinach is wilted.
4. Toss cooked pasta with mushroom and spinach mixture.
5. Sprinkle with nutritional yeast before serving.

Nutritional Info: Calories: 260, Protein: 12g, Fat: 5g, Carbohydrates: 40g

Lentil Pasta with Roasted Vegetables

Gluten-free lentil pasta served with a medley of roasted vegetables.

Preparation Time: 15 minutes, Cooking Time: 25 minutes, Total Time: 40 minutes, serving: 2

Ingredients: 6 oz gluten-free lentil pasta, 1 cup chopped bell peppers, 1 cup chopped zucchini, 1 cup cherry tomatoes (halved), 2 cloves garlic (minced), 2 tablespoons lemon juice.

Direction:

1. Cook lentil pasta according to package instructions.
2. Toss chopped vegetables and minced garlic with lemon juice.
3. Roast in the oven at 400°F for 20 minutes.
4. Serve roasted vegetables over cooked pasta.

Nutritional Info: Calories: 250, Protein: 14g, Fat: 2g, Carbohydrates: 45g

Chickpea Noodle Stir-Fry

Stir-fried chickpea noodles with tofu and mixed vegetables in a savory sauce.

Preparation Time: 20 minutes, **Cooking Time:** 15 minutes, **Total Time:** 35 minutes, serving: 2

Ingredients: 6 oz gluten-free chickpea noodles, 1 block (14 oz) firm tofu (cubed), 1 cup mixed vegetables (such as bell peppers, broccoli, and snap peas), 2 tablespoons soy sauce, 1 tablespoon maple syrup.

Direction:

1. Cook chickpea noodles according to package instructions.
2. In a skillet, stir-fry cubed tofu until golden.
3. Add mixed vegetables and continue to stir-fry until tender.
4. Stir in soy sauce and maple syrup.
5. Serve over cooked chickpea noodles.

Nutritional Info: Calories: 320, Protein: 16g, Fat: 4g, Carbohydrates: 50g

Quinoa Noodle Salad with Avocado Dressing

Cold quinoa noodle salad tossed in a creamy avocado dressing with fresh vegetables.

Preparation Time: 20 minutes' **Cooking Time:** 10 minutes, **Total Time:** 30 minutes, Serving: 2

Ingredients: 6 oz gluten-free quinoa noodles, 1 cup shredded cabbage, 1/2 cup shredded carrots, 1/4 cup sliced almonds, 1 ripe avocado, 2 tablespoons lime juice.

Direction:

1. Cook quinoa noodles according to package instructions. Rinse under cold water and drain.
2. In a bowl, combine noodles with shredded cabbage, shredded carrots, and sliced almonds.
3. In a blender, blend avocado and lime juice until smooth to make the dressing.
4. Pour over the noodle salad and toss to coat.

Nutritional Info: Calories: 280, Protein: 10g, Fat: 10g, Carbohydrates: 40g

Black Bean Noodle Soup

Hearty noodle soup made with gluten-free black bean noodles and vegetables.

Preparation Time: 15 minutes, **Cooking Time:** 25 minutes, **Total Time:** 40 minutes, serving: 2

Ingredients: 4 oz gluten-free black bean noodles, 4 cups vegetable broth, 1 cup chopped mixed vegetables (such as carrots, celery, and onion), 1/2 cup cooked black beans.

Direction:

1. In a medium pot, bring vegetable broth to a boil.
2. Add chopped vegetables and cooked black beans, then simmer for 15 minutes.
3. Add black bean noodles and cook until tender.
4. Serve hot and enjoy immediately.

Nutritional Info: Calories: 240, Protein: 14g, Fat: 2g, Carbohydrates: 45g

Soybean Noodle Salad with Ginger Dressing

Refreshing soybean noodle salad tossed in a zesty ginger dressing with crunchy vegetables.

Preparation Time: 20 minutes, Cooking Time: 5 minutes, Total Time: 25 minutes, serving: 2
Ingredients: 6 oz gluten-free soybean noodles, 1 cup julienned cucumber, 1/2 cup shredded carrots, 1/4 cup chopped peanuts, 2 tablespoons rice vinegar, 1 tablespoon grated ginger.
Direction:
1. Cook soybean noodles according to package instructions. Rinse under cold water and drain.
2. In a bowl, combine noodles with julienned cucumber, shredded carrots, and chopped peanuts.
3. In a separate bowl, whisk together rice vinegar and grated ginger to make the dressing.
4. Pour over the noodle salad and toss to coat.
Nutritional Info: Calories: 290, Protein: 12g, Fat: 10g, Carbohydrates: 40g

Buckwheat Noodles with Spicy Peanut Sauce

Buckwheat noodles served with a spicy peanut sauce and fresh vegetables for a flavorful dish.
Preparation Time: 20 minutes, Cooking Time: 10 minutes, Total Time: 30 minutes, serving: 2
Ingredients: 6 oz gluten-free buckwheat noodles, 1 cup julienned bell peppers, 1/2 cup sliced scallions, 1/4 cup chopped cilantro, 2 tablespoons peanut butter, 1 tablespoon sriracha sauce.
Direction:
1. Cook noodles according to package instructions. Rinse under cold water and drain.
2. In a bowl, combine noodles with julienned bell peppers, sliced scallions, and chopped cilantro.
3. In a separate bowl, mix peanut butter and sriracha sauce to make the spicy peanut sauce.
4. Pour the dressing over the noodles and toss to coat.
Nutritional Info: Calories: 280, Protein: 10g, Fat: 8g, Carbohydrates: 45g

Mung Bean Noodle Stir-Fry with Tofu

Stir-fried mung bean noodles with tofu and colorful vegetables in a savory sauce.
Preparation Time: 20 minutes, Cooking Time: 15 minutes, Total Time: 35 minutes, serving: 2
Ingredients: 6 oz gluten-free mung bean noodles, 1 block (14 oz) firm tofu (cubed), 1 cup mixed vegetables (such as bell peppers, broccoli, and snap peas), 2 tablespoons soy sauce, 1 tablespoon maple syrup.
Direction:
1. Cook mung bean noodles according to package instructions.
2. In a skillet, stir-fry cubed tofu until golden.
3. Add mixed vegetables and continue to stir-fry until tender.
4. Stir in soy sauce and maple syrup.
5. Serve over cooked mung bean noodles.
Nutritional Info: Calories: 320, Protein: 16g, Fat: 4g, Carbohydrates: 50g

Rice Noodle Salad with Sesame Dressing

Cold rice noodle salad tossed in a sesame dressing with fresh vegetables and herbs.

Preparation Time: 20 minutes, Cooking Time: 5 minutes, Total Time: 25 minutes, Serving: 2

Ingredients: 6 oz gluten-free rice noodles, 1 cup shredded lettuce, 1/2 cup sliced cucumber, 1/4 cup chopped fresh cilantro, 2 tablespoons sesame oil, 1 tablespoon rice vinegar.

Direction:

1. Cook rice noodles according to package instructions. Rinse under cold water and drain.

2. In a bowl, combine noodles with shredded lettuce, sliced cucumber, and chopped fresh cilantro.

3. In a separate bowl, whisk together sesame oil and rice vinegar to make the dressing.

4. Pour over the noodle salad and toss to coat.

Nutritional Info: Calories: 280, Protein: 10g, Fat: 10g, Carbohydrates: 40g

Soba Noodle Salad with Ginger Soy Dressing

Cold soba noodle salad tossed in a ginger soy dressing with crunchy vegetables and sesame seeds.

Preparation Time: 20 minutes, Cooking Time: 5 minutes, Total Time: 25 minutes, Serving: 2

Ingredients: 6 oz gluten-free soba noodles, 1 cup shredded cabbage, 1/2 cup shredded carrots, 1/4 cup sliced scallions, 2 tablespoons soy sauce, 1 tablespoon grated ginger, 1 tablespoon sesame seeds.

Direction:

1. Cook soba noodles according to package instructions. Rinse under cold water and drain.

2. In a bowl, combine noodles with shredded cabbage, shredded carrots, and sliced scallions.

3. In a separate bowl, whisk together soy sauce and grated ginger to make the dressing.

4. Pour over the noodle salad and toss to coat.

5. Sprinkle with sesame seeds before serving.

Nutritional Info: Calories: 290, Protein: 12g, Fat: 8g, Carbohydrates: 45g

Buckwheat Noodles with Miso Sauce

Buckwheat noodles served with a savory miso sauce and steamed vegetables for a satisfying meal.
Preparation Time: 20 minutes, Cooking Time: 10 minutes, Total Time: 30 minutes, serving: 2
Ingredients: 6 oz gluten-free buckwheat noodles, 1 cup steamed broccoli florets, 1/2 cup sliced bell peppers, 1/4 cup sliced mushrooms, 2 tablespoons miso paste, 1 tablespoon rice vinegar.
Direction:
1. Cook buckwheat noodles according to package instructions.
2. Steam broccoli florets until tender. I
3. n a bowl, combine cooked noodles with steamed broccoli, sliced bell peppers, and sliced mushrooms. 4. In a separate bowl, mix miso paste and rice vinegar to make the sauce.
5. Pour over the noodles and vegetables, and toss to coat.
Nutritional Info: Calories: 280, Protein: 10g, Fat: 8g, Carbohydrates: 45g

PASTA RECIPES

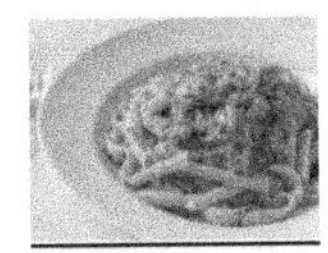

Chickpea Pasta with Tomato Basil Sauce

Gluten-free chickpea pasta served with a flavorful tomato basil sauce.
Preparation Time: 10 minutes, Cooking Time: 20 minutes, Total Time: 30 minutes, serving: 2
Ingredients: 6 oz gluten-free chickpea pasta, 1 cup diced tomatoes, 2 cloves garlic (minced), 1/4 cup chopped fresh basil, 2 tablespoons nutritional yeast.
Direction:
1. Cook chickpea pasta according to package instructions.
2. In a saucepan, sauté minced garlic until fragrant.
3. Add diced tomatoes and cook until softened. Stir in chopped fresh basil and nutritional yeast.
4. Toss with cooked pasta and serve.
Nutritional Info: Calories: 300, Protein: 14g, Fat: 4g, Carbohydrates: 50g

Lentil Pasta with Spinach Pesto

Gluten-free lentil pasta tossed with homemade spinach pesto for a nutritious meal.
Preparation Time: 15 minutes, Cooking Time: 10 minutes, Total Time: 25 minutes, Serving: 2
Ingredients: 6 oz gluten-free lentil pasta, 2 cups fresh spinach leaves, 1/4 cup walnuts, 2 cloves garlic (minced), 2 tablespoons lemon juice.
Direction:

1. Cook pasta according to package instructions.

2. In a food processor, blend spinach, walnuts, garlic, and lemon juice until smooth.

3. Toss cooked pasta with spinach pesto and serve.

Nutritional Info: Calories: 320, Protein: 16g, Fat: 8g, Carbohydrates: 40g

Quinoa Pasta with Roasted Vegetables

Quinoa pasta served with roasted vegetables for a hearty and satisfying meal.

Preparation Time: 15 minutes, Cooking Time: 25 minutes, Total Time: 40 minutes, Serving: 2

Ingredients: 6 oz gluten-free quinoa pasta, 1 cup chopped bell peppers, 1 cup chopped zucchini, 1 cup cherry tomatoes (halved), 2 cloves garlic (minced), 2 tablespoons lemon juice.

Direction:

1. Cook pasta according to package instructions.

2. Toss chopped vegetables and minced garlic with lemon juice.

3. Roast in the oven at 400°F for 20 minutes.

4. Serve roasted vegetables over cooked pasta.

Nutritional Info: Calories: 280, Protein: 12g, Fat: 4g, Carbohydrates: 45g

Soybean Pasta with Mushroom Cream Sauce

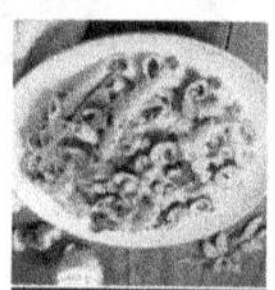

Soybean pasta topped with a creamy mushroom sauce for a decadent dish.

Preparation Time: 15 minutes, Cooking Time: 20 minutes, Total Time: 35 minutes, serving: 2

Ingredients: 6 oz gluten-free soybean pasta, 1 cup sliced mushrooms, 1/2 cup unsweetened almond milk, 2 tablespoons nutritional yeast, 1 tablespoon lemon juice.

Direction:

1. Cook soybean pasta according to package instructions.

2. In a skillet, sauté sliced mushrooms until tender.

3. Stir in almond milk, nutritional yeast, and lemon juice.

4. Simmer until the sauce thickens. Serve over cooked pasta.

Nutritional Info: Calories: 320, Protein: 18g, Fat: 6g, Carbohydrates: 50g

Black Bean Pasta with Avocado Pesto

Black bean pasta served with creamy avocado pesto sauce for a vibrant and nutritious meal.

Preparation Time: 20 minutes, Cooking Time: 10 minutes, Total Time: 30 minutes, serving: 2

Ingredients: 6 oz gluten-free black bean pasta, 1 ripe avocado, 1 cup fresh basil leaves, 1/4 cup pine nuts, 2 cloves garlic (minced).

Direction:

1. Cook black bean pasta according to package instructions.

2. In a food processor, blend avocado, basil leaves, pine nuts, and minced garlic until smooth.
3. Toss cooked pasta with avocado pesto and serve.
Nutritional Info: Calories: 340, Protein: 14g, Fat: 12g, Carbohydrates: 45g

Brown Rice Pasta with Tomato Garlic Sauce

Brown rice pasta topped with a flavorful tomato garlic sauce for a simple yet satisfying dish.
Preparation Time: 10 minutes, Cooking Time: 20 minutes, Total Time: 30 minutes, serving: 2
Ingredients: 6 oz gluten-free brown rice pasta, 1 cup diced tomatoes, 2 cloves garlic (minced), 1/4 cup chopped fresh parsley, 2 tablespoons nutritional yeast.
Direction:
1. Cook brown rice pasta according to package instructions.
2. In a saucepan, sauté minced garlic until fragrant.
3. Add diced tomatoes and cook until softened.
4. Stir in chopped fresh parsley and nutritional yeast.
5. Toss with cooked pasta and serve.
Nutritional Info: Calories: 290, Protein: 10g, Fat: 4g, Carbohydrates: 50g

Chickpea Avocado Pasta

Creamy avocado sauce paired with protein-packed chickpea pasta for a nutritious and satisfying meal.
Preparation Time: 10 minutes, Cooking Time: 10 minutes, Total Time: 20 minutes, serving: 4
Ingredients: 8 oz gluten-free chickpea pasta, 2 ripe avocados, Juice of 1 lemon, 1/4 cup fresh basil leaves, 1/4 cup unsweetened almond milkfv
Directions:
1. Cook chickpea pasta according to package instructions.
2. In a blender, combine ripe avocados, lemon juice, basil leaves, and almond milk until smooth.
3. Toss cooked pasta with the avocado sauce until well coated.
Nutritional Info: Calories: 300, Protein: 12g, Fat: 15g, Carbohydrates: 30g

Tofu Veggie Pasta Primavera

Colorful pasta primavera loaded with vegetables and protein-rich tofu, tossed in a light and refreshing sauce.
Preparation Time: 15 minutes, Cooking Time: 15 minutes, Total Time: 30 minutes, serving: 4
Ingredients: 8 oz gluten-free pasta, 1 block firm tofu, cubed, 2 cups mixed vegetables (such as bell peppers, broccoli, cherry tomatoes), Juice of 1 lime, 2 tablespoons chopped cilantro
Directions:
1. Cook gluten-free pasta according to package instructions.
2. In a skillet, sauté tofu until lightly golden.
3. Add mixed vegetables and cook for about 15 minutes or until tender.

4. Toss cooked pasta with tofu and vegetables.
5. Squeeze lime juice over the pasta and sprinkle with chopped cilantro.
Nutritional Info: Calories: 280, Protein: 14g, Fat: 8g, Carbohydrates: 40g

Lentil Marinara Pasta

Hearty lentil-based marinara sauce served over gluten-free pasta, providing a boost of protein and flavor.

Preparation Time: 10 minutes, Cooking Time: 25 minutes, Total Time: 35 minutes, serving: 4
Ingredients: 8 oz gluten-free pasta, 1 cup dried green lentils, 2 cups marinara sauce, 1/4 cup chopped fresh parsley
Directions:
 1. Cook the lentils according to package instructions and set aside.
2. In a saucepan, combine cooked lentils and marinara sauce.
3. Simmer for 10 minutes over medium low heat.
4. Cook gluten-free pasta according to package instructions.
5. Serve lentil marinara sauce over cooked pasta, garnished with chopped parsley and enjoy.
Nutritional Info: Calories: 320, Protein: 16g, Fat: 4g, Carbohydrates: 55g

Quinoa Pesto Pasta

Nutty quinoa pasta coated in a vibrant homemade pesto sauce, creating a protein-packed and flavorful dish.

Preparation Time: 15 minutes, Cooking Time: 10 minutes, Total Time: 25 minutes, serving: 4
Ingredients: 8 oz gluten-free quinoa pasta, 2 cups fresh basil leave, 1/2 cup raw walnuts, 2 cloves garlic, Juice of 1 lemon, 1/4 cup nutritional yeast
Directions:
1. Cook quinoa pasta according to package instructions.
2. In a food processor, blend basil leaves, walnuts, garlic, lemon juice, and nutritional yeast until smooth. 3. Toss cooked pasta with pesto sauce until well combined.
Nutritional Info: Calories: 340, Protein: 14g, Fat: 15g, Carbohydrates: 45g

Black Bean Lime Pasta

Zesty black bean sauce infused with lime, served over gluten-free pasta for a protein-rich and refreshing dish.

Preparation Time: 10 minutes Cooking Time: 15 minutes, Total Time: 25 minutes, serving: 4
Ingredients: 8 oz gluten-free pasta, 1 can black beans, drained and rinsed, Juice of 2 limes, Zest of 1 lime, 2 tablespoons chopped fresh cilantro
Directions:
1. Cook gluten-free pasta according to package instructions.
2. In a blender, combine black beans, lime juice, and lime zest until smooth.
3. Heat black bean sauce in a saucepan until warmed through.
4. Serve over cooked pasta, garnished with chopped cilantro and enjoy.

Nutritional Info: Calories: 290, Protein: 12g, Fat: 2g, Carbohydrates: 55g

Lentil Pasta with Vegan Alfredo Sauce

Lentil pasta served with a creamy vegan Alfredo sauce made with cauliflower.

Preparation Time: 20 minutes, Cooking Time: 20 minutes, Total Time: 40 minutes, serving: 2

Ingredients: 6 oz gluten-free lentil pasta, 2 cups cauliflower florets, 1/2 cup unsweetened almond milk, 2 tablespoons nutritional yeast, 1 tablespoon lemon juice.

Direction:

1. Cook lentil pasta according to package instructions.
2. Steam cauliflower until tender.
3. In a blender, blend steamed cauliflower with almond milk, nutritional yeast, and lemon juice until smooth.
4. Heat the sauce in a saucepan until warm.
5. Serve over cooked pasta right way and enjoy

Nutritional Info: Calories: 310, Protein: 14g, Fat: 6g, Carbohydrates: 45g

Quinoa Pasta with Roasted Red Pepper Sauce

Quinoa pasta topped with a savory roasted red pepper sauce for a burst of flavor.

Preparation Time: 15 minutes, Cooking Time: 25 minutes, Total Time: 40 minutes, serving: 2

Ingredients: 6 oz gluten-free quinoa pasta, 2 roasted red peppers, 1/4 cup raw cashews, 2 cloves garlic (minced), 1 tablespoon lemon juice.

Direction:

1. Cook quinoa pasta according to package instructions.
2. In a blender bowl, blend roasted red peppers, raw cashews, minced garlic, and lemon juice until smooth.
3. Heat the sauce in a saucepan until warm.
4. Serve sauce over cooked pasta.

Nutritional Info: Calories: 330, Protein: 12g, Fat: 10g, Carbohydrates: 50g

Soybean Pasta with Broccoli Pesto

Soybean pasta tossed with homemade broccoli pesto for a nutritious twist on classic pesto pasta.

Preparation Time: 20 minutes, Cooking Time: 10 minutes, Total Time: 30 minutes, serving: 2

Ingredients: 6 oz gluten-free soybean pasta, 2 cups steamed broccoli florets, 1/4 cup walnuts, 2 cloves garlic (minced), and 2 tablespoons lemon juice.

Direction:

1. Cook soybean pasta according to package instructions.
2. In a food processor, blend steamed broccoli, walnuts, minced garlic, and lemon juice until smooth.
3. Toss cooked pasta with broccoli pesto and serve.

Nutritional Info: Calories: 320, Protein: 14g, Fat: 8g, Carbohydrates: 45g

Black Bean Pasta with Cilantro Lime Sauce

Black bean pasta topped with a zesty cilantro lime sauce for a refreshing and flavorful dish.
Preparation Time: 15 minutes, Cooking Time: 20 minutes, Total Time: 35 minutes, serving: 2
Ingredients: 6 oz gluten-free black bean pasta, 1/2 cup fresh cilantro leaves, 1/4 cup raw cashews, 1 clove garlic (minced), 2 tablespoons lime juice.
Direction:
1. Cook black bean pasta according to package instructions.
2. In a blender, blend cilantro leaves, raw cashews, minced garlic, and lime juice until smooth.
3. Heat the sauce in a saucepan until warm.
4. Serve sauce over cooked pasta.
Nutritional Info: Calories: 340, Protein: 16g, Fat: 10g, Carbohydrates: 50g

CAKE RECIPES

These cake recipes are not only delicious but also packed with protein and free from gluten, dairy, salt, and oil. Enjoy your guilt-free treats!

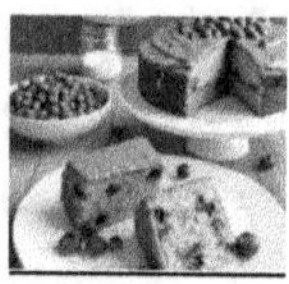

Blueberry Banana Protein Cake

A moist and fluffy cake bursting with blueberries and banana flavor.
Preparation Time: 15 minutes, Cooking Time: 40 minutes, Total Time: 55 minutes, serving: 8
Ingredients: 1 cup gluten-free oat flour, 1/2 cup vanilla protein powder, 1 ripe banana (mashed), 1/4 cup unsweetened almond milk, 1/4 cup maple syrup, 1 cup fresh blueberries, 1 teaspoon baking powder.
Direction:
1. Preheat the oven to 350°F (175°C). In a bowl, protein powder, mix oat flour, and baking powder.
2. Add mashed banana, almond milk, and maple syrup. Stir until combined.
3. Gently fold in blueberries. Pour the batter into a greased cake pan.
4. Bake until a toothpick inserted into the center comes out clean, for about 35 minutes or more.
5. Let it cool before slicing.
Nutritional Info: Calories: 160, Protein: 8g, Fat: 3g, Carbohydrates: 25g

Chocolate Zucchini Protein Cake

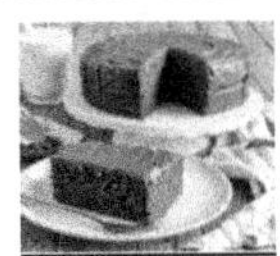

A rich and chocolatey cake with the added goodness of zucchini.

Preparation Time: 20 minutes, Cooking Time: 45 minutes, Total Time: 65 minutes, serving: 8

Ingredients: 1 1/2 cups gluten-free flour, 1/2 cup chocolate protein powder, 1/4 cup unsweetened cocoa powder, 1/4 cup unsweetened applesauce, 1/4 cup almond milk, 1/4 cup maple syrup, 1 cup grated zucchini, 1 teaspoon baking powder.

Direction:

1. Preheat the oven to 350°F (175°C).

2. In a medium mixing bowl, combine flour, cocoa powder, protein powder, and baking powder.

3. Add applesauce, almond milk, and maple syrup. Mix until smooth. Fold in grated zucchini.

4. Pour the batter into a greased cake pan.

5. Bake for about 45 minutes or until a toothpick inserted into the center comes out clean.

6. Let it cool before serving.

Nutritional Info: Calories: 160, Protein: 9g, Fat: 3g, Carbohydrates: 25g

Lemon Raspberry Protein Cake

A tangy lemon cake studded with juicy raspberries.

Preparation Time: 20 minutes, Cooking Time: 35 minutes, Total Time: 55 minutes, serving: 8

Ingredients: 1 1/2 cups almond flour, 1/2 cup vanilla protein powder, zest and juice of 1 lemon, 1/4 cup unsweetened applesauce, 1/4 cup almond milk, 1/4 cup maple syrup, 1 cup fresh raspberries, 1 teaspoon baking powder.

Direction:

1. Preheat the oven to 350°F (175°C). In a bowl, mix almond flour, protein powder, and baking powder. 2. Add lemon zest, lemon juice, applesauce, almond milk, and maple syrup.

3. Stir until well combined and then gently fold in raspberries.

4. Transfer the batter into a greased cake pan.

5. Bake cake for about 31-35 minutes or until golden brown and a toothpick inserted into the center comes out clean.

6. Remove from the oven and let it cool before slicing.

Nutritional Info: Calories: 160, Protein: 8g, Fat: 5g, Carbohydrates: 20g

Peanut Butter Banana Protein Cake

A heavenly combination of peanut butter and banana in a protein-packed cake.

Preparation Time: 15 minutes, Cooking Time: 40 minutes, Total Time: 55 minutes, serving: 8

Ingredients: 1 cup gluten-free oat flour, 1/2 cup vanilla protein powder, 1 ripe banana (mashed), 1/4 cup natural peanut butter, 1/4 cup unsweetened almond milk, 1/4 cup maple syrup, 1 teaspoon baking powder.

Direction:

1. Preheat the oven to 350°F (175°C). In a bowl, combine protein powder, oat flour, and baking powder. 2. Add mashed banana, peanut butter, almond milk, and maple syrup. Mix until smooth.

3. Pour the batter into the prepared cake pan.

4. Bake for 35-40 minutes.

4. Remove from the heat and let it cool before serving. Enjoy!

Nutritional Info: Calories: 160, Protein: 10g, Fat: 4g, Carbohydrates: 20g

Cinnamon Apple Protein Cake

A cozy and comforting cake infused with cinnamon and apples.

Preparation Time: 20 minutes, Cooking Time: 45 minutes, Total Time: 65 minutes Serving: 8

Ingredients: 1 1/2 cups almond flour, 1/2 cup vanilla protein powder, 1 teaspoon ground cinnamon, 1/4 cup unsweetened applesauce, 1/4 cup almond milk, 1/4 cup maple syrup, 1 medium apple (diced), 1 teaspoon baking powder.

Direction:

1. Preheat the oven to 350°F (175°C). In a bowl, mix almond flour, protein powder, cinnamon, and baking powder.

2. Add applesauce, almond milk, and maple syrup. Stir until well combined.

3. Gently fold in diced apple. Pour the batter into a greased cake pan.

4. Bake for 40-45 minutes or until golden brown and a toothpick inserted into the center comes out clean. 5. Let it cool before slicing.

Nutritional Info: Calories: 160, Protein: 9g, Fat: 6g, Carbohydrates: 20g

Chocolate Peanut Butter Protein Cake

A decadent chocolate cake with swirls of creamy peanut butter.

Preparation Time: 25 minutes, Cooking Time: 40 minutes, Total Time: 65 minutes, serving: 8

Ingredients: 1 1/2 cups gluten-free flour, 1/2 cup chocolate protein powder, 1/4 cup unsweetened cocoa powder, 1/4 cup natural peanut butter, 1/4 cup unsweetened almond milk, 1/4 cup maple syrup, 1 teaspoon baking powder.

Direction:

1. Preheat the oven to 350°F (175°C). In a large mixing bowl, combine flour, cocoa powder, protein powder, and baking powder.

2. Add peanut butter, almond milk, and maple syrup.

3. Mix until smooth and then pour the batter into a prepared cake pan.

4. Bake for 35-40 minutes or until a toothpick inserted into the center comes out clean.

5. Remove the cake from heat and let cool before serving.

Nutritional Info: Calories: 160, Protein: 10g, Fat: 5g, Carbohydrates: 20g

Coconut Mango Protein Cake

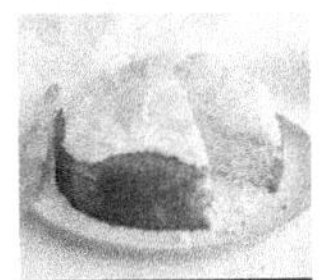

A tropical-inspired cake featuring the flavors of coconut and mango.

Preparation Time: 20 minutes, Cooking Time: 45 minutes, Total Time: 65 minutes, serving: 8

Ingredients: 1 1/2 cups almond flour, 1/2 cup vanilla protein powder, 1/4 cup unsweetened shredded coconut, 1/4 cup unsweetened applesauce, 1/4 cup almond milk, 1/4 cup maple syrup, 1/2 cup diced mango, 1 teaspoon baking powder.

Direction:

1. Preheat the oven to 350°F (175°C). In a bowl, mix almond flour, protein powder, shredded coconut, and baking powder.

2. Add applesauce, almond milk, and maple syrup. Stir until well combined. Fold in diced mango.

3. Pour the cake batter into a greased cake pan.

4. Place the baking pan in oven and bake until golden brown and a toothpick inserted into the center comes out clean, for about 40-45 minute.

5. Remove from the oven and let cool before slicing.

Nutritional Info: Calories: 160, Protein: 9g, Fat: 6g, Carbohydrates: 20g

Pumpkin Spice Protein Cake

A cozy cake infused with warm pumpkin spice flavors.

Preparation Time: 20 minutes, Cooking Time: 40 minutes, Total Time: 60 minutes, serving: 8

Ingredients: 1 1/2 cups gluten-free flour, 1/2 cup vanilla protein powder, 1/2 cup pumpkin puree, 1/4 cup unsweetened applesauce, 1/4 cup almond milk, 1/4 cup maple syrup, 1 teaspoon pumpkin pie spice, 1 teaspoon baking powder.

Direction:

1. Preheat the oven to 350°F (175°C). In a bowl, combine flour, protein powder, pumpkin pie spice, and baking powder.

2. Add pumpkin puree, applesauce, almond milk, and maple syrup. Mix until smooth.

3. Pour the batter into the prepared cake pan and bake for about 40 minutes or until a toothpick inserted into the center comes out clean, 4. Let it cool before serving.

Nutritional Info: Calories: 160, Protein: 8g, Fat: 3g, Carbohydrates: 25g

Strawberry Coconut Protein Cake

A delightful cake infused with the sweetness of strawberries and coconut.

Preparation Time: 20 minutes, Cooking Time: 40 minutes, Total Time: 60 minutes, serving: 8

Ingredients: 1 1/2 cups almond flour, 1/2 cup vanilla protein powder, 1/4 cup unsweetened shredded coconut, 1/4 cup unsweetened applesauce, 1/4 cup almond milk, 1/4 cup maple syrup, 1 cup diced strawberries, 1 teaspoon baking powder.

Direction:

1. Preheat the oven to 350°F (175°C).
2. In a bowl, mix almond flour, protein powder, shredded coconut, and baking powder.
3. Add applesauce, almond milk, and maple syrup and stir until well combined.
4. Gently fold in diced strawberries and pour the batter into a greased cake pan.
5. Bake for 35-40 minutes or until golden brown and a toothpick inserted into the center comes out clean. 6. Let it cool before slicing.

Nutritional Info: Calories: 160, Protein: 9g, Fat: 6g, Carbohydrates: 20g

Cherry Chocolate Protein Cake

A decadent chocolate cake with bursts of sweet cherries in every bite.

Preparation Time: 20 minutes, Cooking Time: 40 Minutes, Total Time: 60 minutes Serving: 8

Ingredients: 1 1/2 cups gluten-free flour, 1/2 cup chocolate protein powder, 1/4 cup unsweetened cocoa powder, 1/4 cup unsweetened applesauce, 1/4 cup almond milk, 1/4 cup maple syrup, 1 cup pitted and chopped cherries, 1 teaspoon baking powder.

Direction:

1. Preheat the oven to 350°F (175°C).
2. In a bowl, combine flour, protein powder, cocoa powder, and baking powder.
3. Add applesauce, almond milk, and maple syrup. Mix until smooth.
4. Gently fold in chopped cherries.
5. Pour the batter into the prepared cake pan.
6. Bake for about 40 minutes or until a toothpick inserted into the center comes out clean.
7. Let it cool before serving.

Nutritional Info: Calories: 160, Protein: 10g, Fat: 4g, Carbohydrates: 20g

Vegan Chocolate Protein Cake

A rich and decadent chocolate cake made without eggs, perfect for vegans and those with egg allergies.

Preparation Time: 15 minutes, Cooking Time: 30 minutes, Total Time: 45 minutes, serving: 8

Ingredients: 1 1/2 cups almond flour, 1/2 cup plant-based chocolate protein powder, 1/4 cup cocoa powder, 1/2 cup maple syrup, 1/4 cup unsweetened applesauce, 1/2 cup unsweetened almond milk, 1 teaspoon baking powder

Directions:

1. Preheat the oven to 350°F (175°C). Grease a cake pan.
2. In a mixing bowl, combine almond flour, protein powder, cocoa powder, maple syrup, applesauce, almond milk, and baking powder. Mix until smooth.
3. Pour the batter into the prepared cake pan and bake until a toothpick inserted into the center comes out clean, for about 30 minutes.
4. Remove the cake from the oven and let it cool before serving.
Nutritional Info: Calories: 200, Protein: 12g, Fat: 8g, Carbohydrates: 25g

Vanilla Protein Cake

A light and fluffy vanilla cake without eggs, enriched with plant-based protein powder.
Preparation Time: 15 minutes, Cooking Time: 35 minutes, Total Time: 50 minutes serving: 8
Ingredients: 1 1/2 cups almond flour, 1/2 cup plant-based vanilla protein powder, 1/4 cup maple syrup, 1/4 cup unsweetened applesauce, 1/2 cup unsweetened almond milk, 1 teaspoon baking powder 1 teaspoon vanilla extract
Directions:
1. Preheat the oven to 350°F (175°C). Grease a cake pan.
2. In a mixing bowl, combine almond flour, protein powder, maple syrup, applesauce, almond milk, baking powder, and vanilla extract. Mix until well combined.
3. Pour the batter into the prepared cake pan and bake for 35 minutes or until golden brown.
4. Remove the cake from the oven and let cool before slicing and serving.
Nutritional Info: Calories: 180, Protein: 10g, Fat: 7g, Carbohydrates: 20g

Vegan Lemon Protein Cake

A tangy and refreshing lemon-flavored cake made without eggs and packed with plant-based protein.
Preparation Time: 15 minutes, Cooking Time: 30 minutes, Total Time: 45 minutes, serving: 8
Ingredients: 1 1/2 cups almond flour, 1/2 cup plant-based vanilla protein powder, Zest and juice of 2 lemons, 1/4 cup maple syrup, 1/4 cup unsweetened applesauce, 1/2 cup unsweetened almond milk1 teaspoon baking powder
Directions:
1. Preheat the oven to 350°F (175°C). Grease a cake pan.
2. In a mixing bowl, combine almond flour, protein powder, lemon zest, lemon juice, maple syrup, applesauce, almond milk, and baking powder. Mix until smooth.
3. Pour the batter into the prepared cake pan and bake for about 30 minutes or until a toothpick inserted into the center comes out clean.
4 Remove from the oven and let it cool before serving.
Nutritional Info: Calories: 190, Protein: 11g, Fat: 7g, Carbohydrates: 20g

Blueberry Protein Cake

A delightful blueberry-infused cake without eggs, bursting with fruity flavors and protein.

Ingredients: 1 1/2 cups almond flour, 1/2 cup plant-based vanilla protein powder, 1 cup fresh or frozen blueberries, 1/4 cup maple syrup, 1/4 cup unsweetened applesauce, 1/2 cup unsweetened almond milk, 1 teaspoon baking powder

Directions:

1. Preheat the oven to 350°F (175°C). Grease a cake pan.

2. In a mixing bowl, combine almond flour, protein powder, blueberries, maple syrup, applesauce, almond milk, and baking powder.

3. Mix until well combined. Pour the batter into the prepared baking pan and bake for about 35 minutes or until golden brown.

4. Let it cool before slicing and serving.

Nutritional Info: Calories: 200, Protein: 12g, Fat: 8g, Carbohydrates: 25g

Coconut Protein Cake

A tropical-inspired cake without eggs, featuring coconut flour and plant-based protein powder.

Preparation Time: 15 minutes, Cooking Time: 40 minutes, Total Time: 55 minutes, serving: 8

Ingredients: 1 cup coconut flour, 1/2 cup plant-based vanilla protein powder, 1/4 cup shredded coconut, 1/4 cup maple syrup, 1/4 cup unsweetened applesauce, 1/2 cup unsweetened almond milk. 1 teaspoon baking powder

Directions:

1. Preheat the oven to 350°F (175°C). Grease a cake pan.

2. In a mixing bowl, combine coconut flour, protein powder, shredded coconut, maple syrup, applesauce, almond milk, and baking powder.

3. Mix mixture until smooth. Pour the batter into the prepared pan and bake for 40 minutes or until a toothpick inserted into the center comes out clean.

4. Let it cool before serving.

Nutritional Info: Calories: 180, Protein: 10g, Fat: 7g, Carbohydrates: 20g

Pumpkin Protein Cake

A cozy and spiced pumpkin cake without eggs, made with plant-based protein powder for extra nutrition.

Preparation Time: 20 minutes, Cooking Time: 45 minutes, Total Time: 65 minutes, serving: 8

Ingredients: 1 1/2 cups almond flour, 1/2 cup plant-based vanilla protein powder, 1 cup pumpkin puree, 1/4 cup maple syrup, 1/4 cup unsweetened applesauce, 1/2 cup unsweetened almond milk, 1 teaspoon pumpkin pie spice1 teaspoon baking powder

Directions:

1. Preheat the oven to 350°F (175°C). Grease a cake pan.

2. In a mixing bowl, combine almond flour, protein powder, pumpkin puree, maple syrup, applesauce, almond milk, pumpkin pie spice, and baking powder.

3. Mix until well combined. Pour the cake batter to the prepared baking pan and bake for 45 minutes or until a toothpick inserted into the center comes out clean.

4. Let it cool before slicing and serving.
Nutritional Info: Calories: 190, Protein: 11g, Fat: 7g, Carbohydrates: 20g

Vegan Banana Protein Cake

A moist and flavorful banana cake without eggs, enhanced with plant-based protein powder.
Preparation Time: 15 minutes, Cooking Time: 35 minutes, Total Time: 50 minutes, serving: 8
Ingredients: 1 1/2 cups almond flour, 1/2 cup plant-based vanilla protein powder, 2 ripe bananas, mashed, 1/4 cup maple syrup, 1/4 cup unsweetened applesauce, 1/2 cup unsweetened almond milk, 1 teaspoon vanilla extract, 1 teaspoon baking powder
Directions:
1. Preheat the oven to 350°F (175°C).
2. Grease a cake pan. In a mixing bowl, combine almond flour, protein powder, mashed bananas, maple syrup, applesauce, almond milk, vanilla extract, and baking powder. Mix until smooth.
3. Pour the batter into the prepared pan and bake for about 35 minutes or until golden brown.
4. Remove from the oven and let it cool before slicing and serving. Enjoy.
Nutritional Info: Calories: 200, Protein: 12g, Fat: 8g, Carbohydrates: 25g

GRAINS AND STARCHES RECIPES

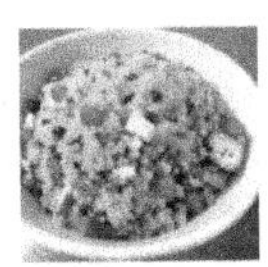

Quinoa Salad

A refreshing salad featuring quinoa, mixed vegetables, and a zesty lemon dressing.
Preparation Time: 15 minutes, Cooking Time: 15 minutes, Total Time: 30 minutes, serving: 4
Ingredients: 1 cup quinoa, rinsed, 2 cups water or vegetable broth, 1 cup cherry tomatoes, halved, 1 cucumber, diced, 1/4 cup red onion, finely chopped. 1/4 cup fresh parsley, chopped, Juice of 1 lemon, 2 tablespoons olive oil (optional)
Directions:
1. In a medium saucepan, bring water or vegetable broth to a boil.
2. Add quinoa, reduce heat to low, and simmer for 15 minutes or until quinoa is tender and liquid is absorbed.
3. Remove the cooked quinoa from heat and let it cool.
4. In a large bowl, combine cooked quinoa, cucumber, cherry tomatoes, parsley and red onion.
5. In a small bowl, whisk together lemon juice and olive oil (if using) to make the dressing.

6. Pour the dressing over the salad and toss to coat. Serve chilled.
Nutritional Info: Calories: 220, Protein: 7g, Fat: 6g, Carbohydrates: 35g

Sweet Potato Hash

A hearty and flavorful dish made with roasted sweet potatoes, bell peppers, and onions.

Preparation Time: 15 minutes, Cooking Time: 25 minutes, Total Time: 40 minutes, serving: 4

Ingredients: 2 large sweet potatoes, diced, 1 red bell pepper, diced, 1 green bell pepper, diced, 1 yellow onion, diced, 2 cloves garlic, minced, 1 teaspoon paprika, 1/2 teaspoon cumin, 1/4 teaspoon black pepper

Directions:

1. Preheat the oven to 400°F (200°C).
2. On a baking sheet, spread diced sweet potatoes, bell peppers, onion, and minced garlic.
3. Sprinkle with paprika, cumin, and black pepper. Toss to coat evenly.
4. Roast in the preheated oven for 20-25 minutes or until vegetables are tender and slightly caramelized. 5. Serve hot as a side dish or topped with avocado slices for a filling meal.

Nutritional Info: Calories: 180, Protein: 4g, Fat: 1g, Carbohydrates: 40g

Brown Rice Stir-Fry

A quick and easy stir-fry made with brown rice, mixed vegetables, and a savory soy sauce.

Preparation Time: 10 minutes, Cooking Time: 20 minutes, Total Time: 30 minutes, serving: 4

Ingredients: 2 cups cooked brown rice, 1 cup mixed vegetables (such as bell peppers, broccoli, carrots), 1/2 cup green peas, 2 cloves garlic, minced, 2 tablespoons low-sodium soy sauce or tamari, 1 tablespoon rice vinegar, 1 tablespoon sesame oil (optional)

Directions:

1. In a large skillet or wok, heat sesame oil (if using) over medium heat.
2. Add minced garlic and cook for a minute until fragrant.
3. Add mixed vegetables and green peas, and stir-fry for 5-7 minutes until tender-crisp.
4. Add cooked brown rice, soy sauce, and rice vinegar to the skillet.
5. Stir well to combine and cook for an additional 3-5 minutes until heated through.
6. Remove from the heat and dive into 4 serving bowl and enjoy.

Nutritional Info: Calories: 220, Protein: 6g, Fat: 3g, Carbohydrates: 45g

Buckwheat Salad

Nutty buckwheat tossed with colorful vegetables and a tangy vinaigrette for a light and satisfying dish.

Preparation Time: 10 minutes, Cooking Time: 15 minutes, Total Time: 25 minutes, serving: 4

Ingredients: 1 cup buckwheat groats, 2 cups water or vegetable broth, 1 cup diced cucumber, 1/2 cup cherry tomatoes, halved, 1/4 cup finely chopped red onion, 1/4 cup chopped fresh parsley, Juice of 1 lemon, 2 tablespoons olive oil

Directions:

1. Rinse buckwheat groats under cold water.
2. In a medium saucepan, bring water or vegetable broth to a boil.
3. Add buckwheat groats, reduce heat to low, and simmer for 10-12 minutes until tender.
4. Remove from heat and let it cool completely.
5. In a large bowl, combine cooked buckwheat, diced cucumber, cherry tomatoes, red onion, and parsley.
6. In a small bowl, whisk together lemon juice and olive oil to make the dressing.
7. Pour the dressing over the salad, toss well to coat and Serve chilled.enjoy!

Nutritional Info: Calories: 240, Protein: 6g, Fat: 8g, Carbohydrates: 35g

Millet Pilaf

A flavorful pilaf made with fluffy millet, sautéed vegetables, and aromatic herbs.

Preparation Time: 10 minutes, Cooking Time: 20 minutes, Total Time: 30 minutes, serving: 4

Ingredients: 1 cup millet, 2 cups vegetable broth, 1 cup diced carrots, 1 cup diced zucchini, 1/2 cup diced bell pepper, 2 cloves garlic, minced, 1 teaspoon dried thyme, 1/2 teaspoon turmeric

Directions:

1. Rinse millet under cold water.
2. In a medium saucepan, bring vegetable broth to a boil.
3. Add millet, reduce heat to low, and simmer for 15-20 minutes until liquid is absorbed and millet is tender.
4. In a separate skillet, sauté diced carrots, zucchini, bell pepper, and minced garlic until vegetables are tender.
5. Stir in cooked millet, dried thyme, and turmeric.
6. Cook for an additional 3-5 minutes until heated through. Serve hot.

Nutritional Info: Calories: 200, Protein: 5g, Fat: 2g, Carbohydrates: 40g

Amaranth Breakfast Porridge

A creamy and nutritious porridge made with amaranth, almond milk, and fresh fruit.

Preparation Time: 5 minutes, Cooking Time: 25 minutes, Total Time: 30 minutes, serving: 4

Ingredients: 1 cup amaranth, 2 cups almond milk, 1/4 cup maple syrup or honey, 1 teaspoon vanilla extract, 1/2 teaspoon cinnamon, Fresh fruit, for serving (such as berries or sliced banana)

Directions:

1. Rinse amaranth under cold water.
2. In a medium saucepan, bring almond milk to a boil.
3. Add amaranth, reduce heat to low, and simmer for 20-25 minutes until creamy and tender, stirring occasionally.
4. Stir in maple syrup or honey, vanilla extract, and cinnamon.

5. Cook for an additional 2-3 minutes. Serve warm topped with fresh fruit.
Nutritional Info: Calories: 220, Protein: 5g, Fat: 4g, Carbohydrates: 40g

Quinoa and Black Bean Bowl

A hearty and nutritious bowl featuring quinoa, black beans, and colorful vegetables.
Preparation Time: 10 minutes, Cooking Time: 15 minutes, Total Time: 25 minutes, serving: 4
Ingredients: 1 cup quinoa, 1 can black beans, drained and rinsed, 1 cup diced tomatoes, 1 avocado, diced, Juice of 1 lime
Directions:
1. Cook quinoa according to package instructions.
2. In a large bowl, combine cooked quinoa, black beans, diced tomatoes, and diced avocado.
3. Squeeze lime juice over the bowl and toss gently to combine. Serve warm or at room temperature.
Nutritional Info: Calories: 240, Protein: 10g, Fat: 8g, Carbohydrates: 35g

Sweet Potato and Chickpea Curry

A flavorful curry made with sweet potatoes, chickpeas, and fragrant spices.
Preparation Time: 15 minutes, Cooking Time: 30 minutes, Total Time: 45 minutes, serving: 4
Ingredients: 2 large sweet potatoes, diced, 1 can chickpeas, drained and rinsed, 1 can coconut milk, 1 cup diced tomatoes, 2 tablespoons curry powder
Directions:
1. In a large pot, combine diced sweet potatoes, chickpeas, coconut milk, diced tomatoes, and curry powder.
2. Bring to a boil, then reduce heat and simmer until sweet potatoes are tender, for about 25-30 minutes.
3. Serve hot over cooked rice or quinoa.
Nutritional Info: Calories: 280, Protein: 10g, Fat: 8g, Carbohydrates: 45g

Roasted Vegetable Medley

A colorful medley of roasted vegetables including potatoes, carrots, and bell peppers.
Preparation Time: 10 minutes, Cooking Time: 30 minutes, Total Time: 40 minutes, serving: 4
Ingredients: 2 large potatoes, diced, 2 carrots, sliced, 1 bell pepper, diced, 1 onion, sliced, 2 tablespoons balsamic vinegar
Directions:
1. Preheat the oven to 400°F (200°C).
2. In a large bowl, toss diced potatoes, sliced carrots, diced bell pepper, and sliced onion with balsamic vinegar until evenly coated.
3. Spread veggies in a single layer on a baking sheet lined with parchment paper.
4. Roast for 25-30 minutes until vegetables are tender and caramelized.
5. Roasted vegetable medley is ready, Serve hot and enjoy.
Nutritional Info: Calories: 220, Protein: 6g, Fat: 2g, Carbohydrates: 45g

Quinoa Salad with Chickpeas

A refreshing salad featuring fluffy quinoa, protein-packed chickpeas, and colorful vegetables.
Preparation Time: 10 minutes, Cooking Time: 15 minutes, Total Time: 25 minutes, serving: 4
Ingredients:, 1 cup quinoa, 1 can chickpeas, drained and rinsed, 1 cup diced cucumber, 1 cup cherry tomatoes, halved, 1/4 cup chopped fresh parsley
Directions:
1. Rinse quinoa under cold water. Cook quinoa according to package instructions.
2. In a large bowl, combine cooked quinoa, chickpeas, diced cucumber, cherry tomatoes, and chopped parsley.
3. Toss gently to combine. Serve chilled or at room temperature.
Nutritional Info: Calories: 220, Protein: 10g, Fat: 4g, Carbohydrates: 35g

Brown Rice and Lentil Bowl

A satisfying bowl featuring hearty brown rice, protein-rich lentils, and a variety of vegetables.
Preparation Time: 10 minutes, Cooking Time: 30 minutes, Total Time: 40 minutes, serving: 4
Ingredients: 1 cup brown rice, 1/2 cup dried green lentils, 2 cups vegetable broth, 1 cup diced bell pepper, 1 cup diced zucchini
Directions:
1. Rinse brown rice and lentils under cold water.
2. In a large pot, combine brown rice, lentils, and vegetable broth.
3. Bring to a boil, then reduce heat and simmer for 25-30 minutes until rice and lentils are tender.
4. In a separate skillet, sauté diced bell pepper and zucchini until tender.
5. Serve cooked rice and lentils in bowls, topped with sautéed vegetables.
Nutritional Info: Calories: 240, Protein: 8g, Fat: 2g, Carbohydrates: 50g

Millet Pilaf with Vegetables

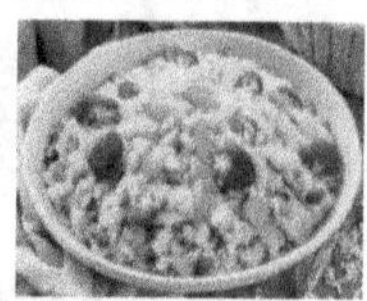

A flavorful pilaf made with fluffy millet, mixed vegetables, and aromatic herbs.
Preparation Time: 10 minutes, Cooking Time: 20 minutes, Total Time: 30 minutes, serving: 4
Ingredients: 1 cup millet, 2 cups vegetable broth, 1 cup diced carrots, 1 cup diced bell pepper, 1/2 cup frozen peas
Directions:
1. Rinse millet under cold water.
2. In a medium saucepan, bring vegetable broth to a boil.
3. Add millet, reduce heat to low, and simmer for 15-20 minutes until liquid is absorbed and millet is tender.
4. In a separate skillet, sauté diced carrots and bell pepper until tender. Stir in frozen peas and cooked millet.
5. Cook for an additional 3-5 minutes until heated through.
6. Serve hot.
Nutritional Info: Calories: 200, Protein: 6g, Fat: 2g, Carbohydrates: 40g

Buckwheat Breakfast Bowl

A nourishing breakfast bowl featuring nutty buckwheat, creamy almond milk, and fresh fruit.
Preparation Time: 5 minutes, Cooking Time: 15 minutes, Total Time: 20 minutes, serving: 2
Ingredients:, 1/2 cup buckwheat groats, 1 cup almond milk, 1/4 cup chopped almonds, 1 ripe banana, sliced
Directions:
1. Rinse buckwheat groats under cold water.
2. In a small saucepan, bring almond milk to a boil.
3. Add buckwheat groats, reduce heat to low, and simmer for 12-15 minutes until buckwheat is tender and liquid is absorbed.
4. Divide cooked buckwheat into bowls.
5. Top with sliced banana and chopped almonds. Serve warm.
Nutritional Info: Calories: 250, Protein: 8g, Fat: 6g, Carbohydrates: 45g